Beating
Chronic
Lyme

New ideas to conquer an enigma
that has left so many wounded

Dr Kevin Conners, DC

Beating Chronic LYME

Dr. Kevin Conners
Fellowship in Integrative Cancer Therapy
Fellowship in Anti-Aging, Regenerative, and Functional Medicine
American Academy of Anti-Aging Medicine

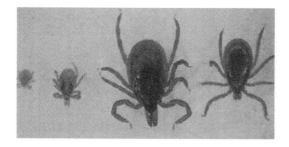

From left to right: Larvae, Nymph, Female, Male Tick

Tick in Nymph stage is the size of a poppy seed.

Beating Chronic LYME

Forward

I used to live in the woods. My wife and four children at the time purchased 280 acres in Wisconsin and basically lived off the land. We grew most of our own food, were 'off grid' as we produced our own electricity through solar panels, and had to pump our water by hand. It was certainly a different way of life that prepared us for missionary work in Mexico.

It was 1997 and at the time I had begun hearing about Lyme disease being a tick-born disorder. I had never seen a deer tick before moving to our 'little house in the big woods' but one thing was for certain – we had plenty of deer. They were as populous as the mosquitoes.

To make a long story short, both my oldest daughter and I had contracted Lyme during our three year stay. I experienced the violent sickness of acute Lyme as well as a beautiful bulls-eye rash that made the diagnosis easy. I took just 3 days of antibiotics and since that was just the second time that I had ever taken a prescription medication in my life, they eradicated the disease effectively.

My daughter on the other hand wasn't so fortunate. She never had an acute illness and we never saw any rash therefore we didn't catch the disease until it had advanced to Chronic Lyme Disease (CLD). This was my first experience (that I know) with CLD and drove me to find answers in a sea of medical disbelief.

Since these first encounters with Lyme, I have cared for thousands of acute and chronic Lyme patients. This short book contains my current line of thinking on the care and cure of chronic Lyme. It is a slippery disease and I am constantly learning (with each new patient I face) how to better care for those suffering the effects of this. Don't believe anyone who says they have all the answers as that just doesn't exist. I pray that this short book will help someone desperate for a solution.

Beating Chronic LYME

Chapter One – Defining a Misunderstood Disease

Chapter Two – Giving the "Little Bugger" Credit

Chapter Three – Understanding the Immune Response

Chapter Four – Thoughts on Solutions

Chapter Five – My Personal Philosophy

"Don't become a mere recorder of facts, but try to penetrate the mystery of their origin."
Ivan Pavlov

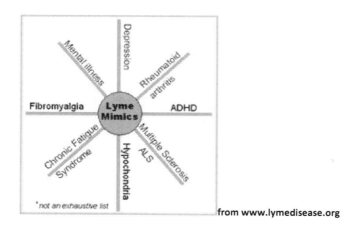

Preface and Disclaimer: I cannot take credit for what's in this book. The Book of Ecclesiastes states, "What has been will be again, what has been done will be done again; there is nothing new under the sun." (Ecc 1:9) Information contained here is simply a small piece of 28 years of practice experience learning from other doctors who've paved my way, scientists dedicated to finding answers, and patients who share their stories. This is in no way a 'complete work', it is a start; I am not an Infectious Disease Specialist, I am a chiropractor with advanced training in neurology, integrative cancer, anti-aging and functional medicine, nutrition, etc. I am simply attempting to convey information and opinion; this is not a substitute for medical care. Any and all information in this book is NOT a substitute for standard medical care. Please consult your physician before considering any information in this book. This book is an opinion, not a protocol, it is the reader's responsibility to seek appropriate medical care and to understand that this book does not suggest or imply that treating cancer is anything but reserved for appropriate medical establishments. Please see the full disclaimer at the end of this book.

Dr. Kevin Conners
Fellowship in Integrative Cancer Therapy
Fellowship in Anti-Aging, Regenerative, and Functional Medicine
American Academy of Anti-Aging Medicine

Beating Chronic LYME

Chapter One

Defining a Misunderstood Disease

"~~Russia~~ (Lyme) is a riddle wrapped in a mystery inside an enigma."

Winston Churchill

What is it?

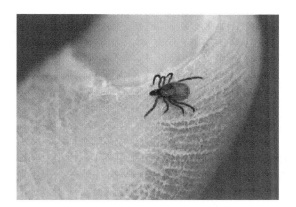

There is argument in the medical community whether chronic Lyme even exists. The general stance by most state medical boards is that it doesn't and that no doctor may treat such figments of imagination. Those who suffer from it have been told to seek psychiatric help, put on antidepressants, and have been made to feel like they are hypochondriacs. But we know that it is real! Chronic Lyme Disease (CLD) is a seriously complex, multi-system, inflammatory, autoimmune disease that is triggered by the bacterial lipoproteins (BLPs) produced by the spiral-shaped bacteria of the family called Borrelia. Though acute Lyme may be acknowledged by most doctors as one cannot continue to ignore the evidence of an identifiable bacterial infection, the inability of antibiotics to kill it after a period of time is what is in question.

The problem is that the Borrelia family of parasites (currently over 90 by count) is difficult to detect, isolate, grow, and study in the laboratory, so our technical knowledge of this pathogen is poor and misunderstood. The disease can affect every tissue and every major organ system in the body. Clinically, it can appear as a chronic arthralgia (joint pain), fibromyalgia (fibrous connective tissue and muscle pain), chronic fatigue, immune dysfunction and as neurological disease. CLD may even be fatal in severe cases depending on severity and the organ being attacked. However, I don't believe that anyone has ever had CLD listed as their cause of death. Why? Because the Borrelia bacteria causes other named diseases which will be explained in Chapter Two.

The diagnosis of Lyme disease *should be* primary based upon clinical evidence but time and time again I see patients who are unable to receive a necessary, immediate antibiotic until labs are run. There is currently no perfect, laboratory test that is definitive for Lyme disease. Most tests will still give false negative results – meaning the patient is told they are fine and they are NOT. Physicians not familiar with the complex clinical presentation (could I say MOST) of Lyme disease frequently misdiagnose it as other disorders. Left untreated in its acute phase, it (the spirochete) can become an antigen in a variety of autoimmune disorders such as: Fibromyalgia or Chronic Fatigue Immune Dysfunction Syndrome (CFIDS), Multiple Sclerosis, Lupus, Parkinson's, Alzheimer's, Rheumatoid Arthritis, Motor Neuron Disease (ALS, Amyotrophic Lateral Sclerosis -Lou Gehrig's disease), Multiple Chemical Sensitivity Syndrome (MCS) and numerous other psychiatric disorders such as depression and anxiety.

Though Lyme disease is a familiar name to most people, their knowledge of it is often limited. Unfortunately, your local medical community may know even less. There have been numerous reports in the media about it in the United States over the past 25 years about small deer ticks transmitting bacteria called *Borrelia burgdorferi*. Frequently mentioned is the bulls-eye skin rash that develops following the bite of an infected tick. The disease can begin with flu-like symptoms that progress to a chronic, debilitating disorder.

I wrote this book as an urgent warning for everyone. Acute Lyme disease, left untreated, will become CLD which is devastating the lives of hundreds of thousands of individuals (most never suspecting Lyme as the cause of their disease) and we are all at risk. Most are misdiagnosed and mistreated. In many cases of Lyme disease, a correct diagnosis doesn't occur until after several months or more often many years of suffering with the disease. Even if the blood tests were perfect, waiting a week for the results may be too late! By then it may have caused severe illness, disability and permanent damage. The disease is widespread and the prevalence is significantly higher than reported by health officials.

There are some key factors that exist in the medical community regarding Lyme disease; they go a long way in explaining why CLD is often misdiagnosed and mistreated however, possibly the greatest reason that acute Lyme becomes Chronic Lyme Disease (CLD) is the following criteria (hoops) that standard medical doctors must jump through to legally diagnose:

"Internationally recognized criteria for the diagnosis of Lyme borreliosis are based upon stringent interpretation of serological tests for specific antibodies to B. burgdorferi sensu lato. The criteria recommended in the USA (from the Centers for Disease Control and Prevention), Europe (i.e. MiQ 20-00 Germany) and the UK are:

- Serum samples for the detection of antibodies to B. burgdorferi should be analyzed by a two-test procedure:

  - a sensitive screening test (e.g. ELISA or IFA). All samples judged to be reactive or equivocal in the screening test should then be confirmed by
  - a Western blot for antibodies to specific B. burgdorferi antigens. The Western blot should only be used in succession with an ELISA or IFA test. Detailed interpretive criteria for Western blots differ between Europe and the USA, to take into account differences in the geographic distribution of the infecting genospecies.

These serological criteria are used for the laboratory diagnosis of Lyme borreliosis by the HPA Lyme Borreliosis Specialist Diagnostic Service at the HPA South-East Regional Laboratory, Southampton." (1)

The evidence continues to mount that Chronic Lyme Disease (CLD) exists and must be addressed by the medical community if solutions are to be found.(2) Thirty-four percent of a "population-based, retrospective cohort study in Massachusetts" were found to have arthritis or recurrent arthralgias, neurocognitive impairment, and neuropathy or myelopathy, a mean of 6 years after treatment for Lyme disease (LD) (3). Sixty-two percent of "a cohort of 215 consecutively treated LD patients in Westchester County" were found to have arthralgias, arthritis, and cardiac or neurologic involvement with or without fatigue a mean of 3.2 years after treatment (4).

According to Cameron (2), "There is no objective way to rule out an active infection. Lab tests that can be very helpful in confirming a clinical diagnosis of Lyme disease (such as the ELISA and Western blot tests) are not useful in determining whether the infection has been adequately treated. Common LD symptoms such as Bell's palsy, erythema migrans rash, meningitis, arthritis, or heart block, which are included in the current surveillance definitions, can be useful in "ruling in" Lyme disease, but the absence or disappearance of these symptoms cannot "rule out" an ongoing infection. A population-based, retrospective cohort study of individuals with a history of LD revealed that they were significantly more likely to have joint pain, memory impairment, and poor functional status due to pain than persons without a history of LD, even though there were no signs of objective findings on physical examination or neurocognitive testing (5). Two recent mouse studies revealed that spirochetes persist despite antibiotic therapy and that standard diagnostic tests are not able to detect their presence (6, 7). In sum, there are no clinical or laboratory markers that identify the eradication of the pathogen.

1. "Unorthodox and Unvalidated Laboratory Tests in the Diagnosis of Lyme Borreliosis and in Relation to Medically Unexplained Symptom", Duerden, B.I., UK Health Protection Agency Official Report on Lyme Disease
2. Proof That Chronic Lyme Disease Exists, Daniel J. Cameron, Department of Medicine, Northern Westchester Hospital, Mt.

Kisco, NY 10549, USA, Received 11 December 2009; Accepted 26 March 2010

3. *N. A. Shadick, C. B. Phillips, E. L. Logigian, et al., "The long-term clinical outcomes of Lyme disease. A population-based retrospective cohort study," Annals of Internal Medicine, vol. 121, no. 8, pp. 560–567, 1994.*

4. *E. S. Asch, D. I. Bujak, M. Weiss, M. G. E. Peterson, and A. Weinstein, "Lyme disease: an infectious and postinfectious syndrome," Journal of Rheumatology, vol. 21, no. 3, pp. 454–461, 1994.*

5. *N. A. Shadick, C. B. Phillips, O. Sangha, et al., "Musculoskeletal and neurologic outcomes in patients with previously treated Lyme disease," Annals of Internal Medicine, vol. 131, no. 12, pp. 919–926, 1999.*

6. *E. Hodzic, S. Feng, K. Holden, K. J. Freet, and S. W. Barthold, "Persistence of Borrelia burgdorferi following antibiotic treatment in mice," Antimicrobial Agents and Chemotherapy, vol. 52, no. 5, pp. 1728–1736, 2008. View at Publisher · View at Google Scholar · View at PubMed*

7. *H. Yrjänäinen, J. Hytönen, K.-O. Söderström, J. Oksi, K. Hartiala, and M. K. Viljanen, "Persistent joint swelling and borrelia-specific antibodies in Borrelia garinii-infected mice after eradication of vegetative spirochetes with antibiotic treatment," Microbes and Infection, vol. 8, no. 8, pp. 2044–2051, 2006. View at Publisher · View at Google Scholar · View at PubMed*

CLD is frequently misdiagnosed

I don't believe that it is just my office that attracts people who have had Physicians frequently overlook cases of Lyme disease simply because they don't know the complex pathogenesis of the disease. Nearly every week I see someone telling me a story of how they believed they had an acute Lyme attack, had evidence of a tick bite and experienced typical symptoms suggesting Lyme, only to engage in an argument with their primary doctor and leave untreated. Lyme disease may cause well over 100 different symptoms; the common arthralgia (joint pain) is a CLD symptom that most physicians are familiar with; however, it is only one of many symptoms caused by Lyme disease.

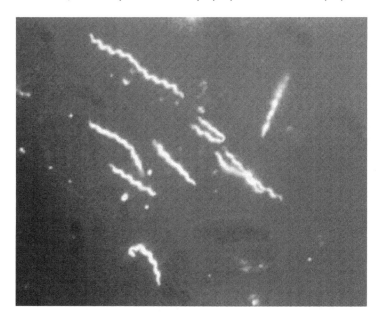

CLD Spirochetes

"The evidence continues to mount that Chronic Lyme Disease (CLD) exists and must be addressed by the medical community if solutions are to be found. Four National Institutes of Health (NIH) trials validated the existence and severity of CLD. Despite the evidence, there are physicians who continue to deny the existence and severity of CLD, which can hinder efforts to find a solution." (1)

Understand that one can get Lyme disease multiple times. I am a perfect example; I had and cured acute Lyme disease years ago and then was re-infected by a new, acute Lyme bite. In a study that revealed this with data proving that Lyme can be killed with antibiotics if caught in the "bacterial phase", the author states, "Our data provide compelling evidence that courses of antibiotics that are recommended by Infectious Disease Society of America regularly cure early Lyme disease," said Nadelman, a professor of medicine in the division of infectious diseases at New York Medical College in Valhalla, in a telephone interview. "When people have early Lyme disease again, it's likely due to a new infection due to a new tick bite." (2)

Most doctors don't know that laboratory tests are often useless and misleading – some reports suggest a 60-70% false negative rate! The laboratory isolation and identification of borrelia is rarely successful; and no clinical test currently exists that can definitively diagnose Lyme disease with 100% accuracy. This is why a diagnosis of Lyme disease should be heavily based upon clinical information such as history, symptoms, and response to therapy. There is an art to medicine when dealing with Lyme disease and experienced physicians must use keen clinical skills and judgment as well as cutting edge diagnostic techniques such as Applied Kinesiology when dealing with suspect Lyme disease patients.

I liken modern medicine to auto mechanics. There was a time when an astute mechanic could listen to an engine and declare that the first lifter was sticking. Now we have become so sophisticated that without a $20,000 computer it is nearly impossible to accurately diagnose a car's problem. Though mechanics may have retained much of their working knowledge, it appears that most physicians have not. They seem lost without an MRI, CT scan, and lab work. I am not saying that there isn't great information derived from such advanced tools, but god, old-fashioned diagnostic skills can become forgotten. Therefore, clinical diagnosis (and the competence to do so) should be made based on the physician's knowledge of the disease. (3)

If a physician is going to rely solely on laboratory tests to confirm a diagnosis of Lyme, they will be wrong more often than right! Most MDs don't know that borrelia produce a large variety of toxic bacterial lipoproteins (BLPs) and they aren't familiar with the way these BLPs cause the symptoms of the disease. The criteria being used to report Lyme disease by physicians is often set by state health officials and is often based upon the rigid criteria established by the Center for Disease Control and Prevention (CDC). This CDC criterion was established for an epidemiological survey, which was designed to study the distribution of Lyme disease. The two-step method of the CDC uses a screening immunoassay for all patients followed by a more sensitive and specific Western blot only if the screening test was positive. Unfortunately, this approach was originally intended for *surveillance* of Lyme disease in potentially asymptomatic patients, not for diagnostic purposes in patients with symptoms that are potentially related to Lyme disease. This criterion was not intended to be used as a standard for the clinical diagnosis of Lyme disease; the CDC has clearly stated this. Unfortunately, ignorant health officials and physicians continue to use these criteria for the clinical diagnosis of Lyme disease.

1. *Interdiscip Perspect Infect Dis. 2010;2010:876450. doi: 10.1155/2010/876450. Epub 2010 May 25., Proof that chronic lyme disease exists. Cameron DJ. Source: Department of Medicine, Northern Westchester Hospital, Mt. Kisco, NY 10549, USA.*
2. *Chronic Lyme Disease Discounted as New Infections BlamedBy Michelle Fay Cortez - Nov 14, 2012 11:00 PM CT*
3. *"The laboratory diagnosis of Lyme borreliosis: guidelines from the Canadian Public Health Laboratory Network", Canadian Public Health Network, Can. J. Infect. Dis. Med. Microbiol. 18: 145-148, 2007.*

Problems with Misdiagnosis

The following description of a married marital couple illustrates the potential seriousness and persistence of increasingly common Lyme and its co-infections and the absolute necessity to receivev a proper diagnosis. These cases are described by Virginia T. Sherr, M.D., a psychiatrist in private practice in Holland, PA. These, as well as case histories similar (possibly yours) demonstrate immediate need for intensive education of all physicians and the public about the risks posed by tick-borne infections. Experiences of these 2 patients demonstrate necessity for accurate epidemiological reporting of all such vector-borne diseases. Of the titled infections, only Lyme and ehrlichiosis are on the Center of Diseases Control's list of Officially Reportable Diseases.

Descriptions of the patients' symptoms:

Mr. W's infection— unrecognized chronic Lyme disease initiated a medical controversy

"Mr. W, an active 76-year-old man (1996) upon his first ever visit to a psychiatrist's office, needed evaluation due to marked changes in his personality. Careful history-taking revealed that he had experienced a rectangular dark red rash on 1 ankle (otherwise asymptomatic) for several weeks circa June 1996. By late that summer, he had gradually developed uncharacteristic and inappropriate outbursts of extreme irritability, altered gait, loss of direction sense, evening chills, episodic daytime sleep urgency, pronounced executive memory loss and variable loss of recent memory. Neurologic and psychiatric workups ensued. In September 1996, his neurologist diagnosed Lyme disease (LYD) when an enzyme-linked immunosorbent assay blood test revealed a positive IgG of 2.63. Doxycycline 100 mg twice daily was begun. Mr. W became less symptomatic, his rages abated, and his memory improved. Another specialist, however, questioned accuracy of the diagnosis, terminating the antibiotic after 2 weeks. Axillary lymphadenopathy remained unexplained.

As June 1997 approached, Mr. W's sore left knee was visibly swollen. Nine months after original diagnosis, he also had developed balance problems, strange, shifting, tender, acutely painful areas on his scalp and feet, and a highly distracting, tingling sensation on the tip of his nose. His family physician examined him and confirmed the original diagnosis of persistent, neuro-Lyme disease.

On 6/3/97, prior to antibiotic treatment, Mr. W suddenly experienced an episode of violent, seizure-like shaking of his entire body, during which he did not lose consciousness. (1,2) There were no urinary tract or other symptoms. His LYD Western Blot (WB) test (7/9/97) revealed 4 highly significant positive IgG bands plus another: an equivocal band on the same WB test for immune antibodies relating to the causative spirochete, Borrelia burgdorferi (Bb).(3)

Gradually improving but still symptomatic following several months of oral antibiotics, Mr. W's WB immune response increased to show 6 positive, significant, IgG antibody bands against Bb. (4/8/98). Intensive antibiotic treatment consisted of concomitant oral cefuroxime axetil, cefixime and doxycycline 100 mg three times per day. His knee swelling totally subsided. Later, receiving azithromycin alone, the patient's irritability, disorientation, cognitive problems, and all but 2 other symptoms resolved. He retained his intense need for lengthy daytime naps despite sound nighttime sleep and he experienced episodic afternoon chills despite normal body temperature. He had episodes of dark urine. Diagnostically, however, physicians did not consider babesiosis early on.

When waves of daytime narcoleptic-like sleep attacks and chilliness intensified during evening hours, despite the use of antibiotics, and Mr. W complained that winter's coldness depressed him, he was further evaluated. On 3/26/98, his blood tested positive with a 1:512 indirect fluorescent antibody (IFA) titer for Babesia microti at BBI (now

"Specialty") Laboratory. His *B microti* polymerase chain reaction (PCR) was also positive (7/7/98) at Medical Diagnostic Laboratories (MDL). Treatment rounds of anti-protozoan medications atovaquone (Mepron) and azithromycin (Zithromax) were undertaken for babesiosis.

Overview of the husband's follow-up laboratory findings and treatment of babesiosis

Fifteen months into treatment by a LYD specialist (4) for chronic babesiosis and LYD, the patient's *B microti* PCR turned negative but his *B burgdorferi* DNA (PCR at MDL) was positive. Mepron was stopped and antibiotic treatment continued. When symptoms resurged in approximately 1 year concomitant with an increasing Human Monocytic Ehrlichiosis (HME) titer, restarting his doxycycline (9/27/00) provided general relief and resolution of lymphadenopathy. However, by April 2001, Mr. W's disorientation, chilliness and sleep urgency intensified once more. His PCR for *B microti* DNA again returned positive, as did his WB for the same organism (MDL).

Because of the positive direct blood test for *B microti* DNA, clinical improvement from LYD symptoms, and the first time fully negative Lyme IgG WB, new emphasis began on re-treatment of chronic babesiosis (5/02). Mr. W received the anti-malarial, Malarone (atovaquone with proquanil), but he also was given a course of dirithromycin (Dynabac) to maintain suppression of likely persistent subclinical borrelial infection. Rationale was that presence of co-infections greatly magnified severity of each. Eventual return of original Lyme disorientation and knee symptoms, however, unveiled resurgences of Lyme WB IgG antibodies (now up to 7 significant bands, 1/30/02—IGeneX Lab) and at MDL, an increase to 3 Babesia antibody bands.(5) At no time did Mr. W need psychotropic medications, other than the stimulant described below.

Interpretation of Mr. W's experience with babesiosis

Mr.W had multiple cycles of treatment with antimicrobial medications (atovaquone, azithromycin, and a combination of atovaquone and proquanil) throughout 4 years with much improvement in memory, affect and general health. Both direct PCR evidence of *Babesia* infection and indirect Babesia tests (increasingly positive antibodies) remained confirmatory of his having active chronic babesiosis. When anti-babesia medication lapsed, there were returns to lab and clinical abnormalities.

Persistent daytime sleep urgency despite lengthy antimicrobial treatment, and 6 PM daily chills, may have been residual signs of chronic babesiosis. However, the narcolepsy-like symptom cannot totally be separated from LYD. Direct evidence of both Lyme and babesiosis was still present by positive DNA testing in April 2001 and by increasing antibodies to both in January 2002. Recent intensification of his sleep attacks coincident with current absence of anti-protozoan treatments suggests babesiosis causation. Modafinil (Provigil) 200 mg twice daily greatly improved his wakefulness. Recent developments of positive PCRs for mycoplasma, HHV-6 and a newly developed mild sleep apnea imply possibility of additional causations of his increasing sleep urgency. Of significance, likewise, there are now diminished blood levels of androstenedione, ACTH, ADH and MSH and increased osmolality—a syndrome frequently seen following illness due to chronic neurotoxic diseases (6) such as Lyme disease and a methicillin-resistant coagulase-negative naso-pharyngeal infection that was diagnosed and treated.

Mrs. W's infections, laboratory findings and treatment

Mrs. W's initially unrecognized tick-borne disease manifested neurologically and muscularly. A 66-year-old gardener, she accompanied her husband for evaluation. She described a medically-observed, ring-shaped red rash on the skin of one forearm (1990). At least 3 other similar rashes were observed in the years surrounding that event—2 had the appearance of a "bull's eye." Seronegative by the ELISA and conventional WB tests, and having no "flu-like symptoms," Mrs. W was not considered by specialists to have a treatable tick-borne disease (TBD) until 1997 when chronic neuroborreliosis with multi-system Lyme involvement was diagnosed clinically by her family doctor. Among many symptoms were profound sense of coldness, entire bodily weakness and generalized, painful, severe muscular spasms, cardiac laboring and arrhythmias, waves of painful aural, visual, and touch hypersensitivities, aphonia, a maxillary bone-gum fistula, bradypnea, impatience, multiple sclerosis-like neurological symptoms, chills, and losses of visual acuity. Ocular examination showed a punctate retinal hemorrhage. She appeared on the verge of imminent collapse. Babesiosis originally was not a suspected co-infection.

Mrs. W's intensive, 8 months' treatment with intravenous (IV) medications—ceftriaxone followed by IV cefotaxime for treatment of the persistently severe late-stage neuro-LYD symptoms, led to a steady improvement. Attempts to truncate treatment resulted in memory losses and return of muscle pain. She also had received doxycycline 100 mg three times daily for newly resurgent Human Monocytic Ehrlichiosis. Her neurological symptoms, restless legs syndrome, cardiac laboring, unrelenting muscle pains, and generalized weakness slowly lessened but recurred with each attempt to discontinue antibiotics.

Gradual relief continued until January 1998 when treatment for LYD suddenly appeared to falter. While still on IV cefotaxime, symptoms intensified with multiple daily waves of skin flushing, sweating, cardiac arrhythmias, pricking, burning, or searing cutaneous pains, weakness, chills, painful muscle spasms, generalized itching, severe hyperacusis, blurred vision, parched lips, impatience, irritability, clumsiness, insomnia, and exquisite hypersensitivity to touch. Episodic scalp and facial sweating occurred in waves with concomitant late afternoon malaise and episodic chills.

IFA blood tests for *Babesia* then revealed a high titer of 1:512 (BBI). However, Mrs. W was afebrile, with subnormal oral temperatures (7) usually ranging from 95.7 to 97.0º F Historically, the patient had experienced unexplained blood losses during 2 otherwise uneventful elective surgeries, one preceding and one following this crisis time by several years, although other routine hemograms were consistently normal. Oral iron (300-600 mg/day) restored her postoperative Hgb from 8% to 14.5% each occasion but did not stop profound malaise and episodic chilliness.

Overview of the wife's laboratory findings and treatment of babesiosis

Mrs. W's initial *Babesia* antibody test, negative (1/05/98), was first done many months after IV and oral treatments, including azithromycin, were started to treat her chronic neuroborreliosis (July 1997). She still was being treated for both LYD and ehrlichiosis and symptoms from these were resolving slowly when daily waves of malaise dramatically escalated, incapacitating her in her 8th month of IV antibiotic treatment. Babesiosis was reconsidered diagnostically.

On 3/26/98, IFA tests for *B microti* done at BBI Laboratory revealed the above-mentioned strongly positive babesiosis titer. *Babesia* PCR blood DNA testing also was positive a year later (March 1999, IGeneX Laboratory), following partial treatment with atovaquone and azithromycin for her newly recognized chronic babesiosis.(8,9) Thus, three independent laboratories confirmed positive testing for *B microti*. In addition, a Fluorescent in situ Hybridization (FISH) test (IGeneX) was positive for fluorescing merozoite ring forms of *Babesia* piroplasms. MDL Lab also found Mrs. W's PCR test for Lyme DNA positive (11/8/99). Of additional interest, when the 2 other known diseases were diminished by treatment, there was a return of a variety of symptoms. Ehrlichiosis antibody (HME IgM) titers were then found to have risen to 1:160 (November 1999, IGeneX Lab). Symptomatic relief followed re-treatment with doxycycline. In April 2001, Mrs. W again had evidence of babesiosis via a positive *B microti* WB (MDL). Her Lyme tests now showed 3 significant positive bands on the IgM WB—a known marker for *chronic* as well as acute LYD. (10)

Interpretation of Mrs. W's Experience

Intensive treatment for babesiosis and Lyme disease over the span of 4 years returned a handicapped Mrs. W to much improved capacity.

However, her life still has to be managed around 2–9 milder daily waves of likely *Babesia*-provoked symptoms. Chills subsided *temporarily* when atavoquone and zithromycin were prescribed. Later, as with her husband, a nasopharyngeal culture was positive for the newly discovered neurotoxin-former, methicillin-resistant, coagulase negative*Staphylococcus epidermidis* that had contributed to her discomfort prior to its specific antibiotic treatment.(6)

Summary of Both Cases

Mr. and Mrs. W, both of whom have documented cases of chronic tick-borne illnesses, including babesiosis, have lived in Pennsylvania most of their lives. Lesions appeared after gardening in their wooded, deer-populated, backyard north of Philadelphia. Neither spouse has been re-exposed to ticks.

Both partners have had normal MRIs. However, single-photon emission computed tomography (SPECT) scans of their brains revealed "global heterogeneous hypoperfusion" compatible with impact of noxious influences upon cerebral circulation, cited by the radiologist as likely related to the LYD of each.(11) For one partner microscopically fluorescing intra-erythrocytic parasites were found in 3 widely spaced evaluations. Neither mate had the acute babesia signs of splenic enlargement or severe hypotension.(12) They were not tested for urinary hemolysis until after atavoquone treatment (13) when these tests were negative. Diagnoses of babesiosis eventually helped to partially explain the inability of both patients to recover fully despite intensive treatment for LYD. Treatment then, for *B microti* infection, sufficiently restored both partners so that they can pursue physical and cognitive activities, although neither is asymptomatic or fully recovered.

Conclusions

Lack of general medical awareness of the presence, persistence, and severity of these widely epidemic and backyard-located, spirochetal, rickettsial and protozoan infections caused significant delay in the treatment of this couple. The delay prolonged their illnesses resulting in severe discomfort and long-term disabilities. Early recognition and medical intervention could have prevented much of the ultimate persistence of their infections.(14)

Official recording of *all* vector-borne illnesses in humans needs to be instituted, in order to bring to universal awareness the true scope of the epidemic and the necessity of proper differentiation and treatment of such infections as Lyme disease, ehrlichiosis, and babesiosis."

(From Two Detailed Case Histories Involving Patients with Co-Infections, by VIRGINIA T. SHERR, M.D., MAY, 2004)

1. *Benach JL, Coleman JL, Habicht GS, et al. Serological evidence for simultaneous occurrences of Lyme disease and babesiosis. J Infect Dis 1985 Sept;152(3):473-477.*

2. *Clark IA, Jacobson LS. Do babesiosis and malaria share a common disease process? Ann Trop Med Parasitol 1998 Jun;92(4):483-8.*

3. *Harris NS. The laboratory's role in the diagnosis of Lyme disease. In: Folds JD, Nakamura RM, eds. Clinical Diagnostic Immunology: Protocol in Quality Assurance and Standardization. Malden, Mass: Blackwell Science, 1998:362-382.*

4. *Bach GP. Antibiotics and atovaquone for Lyme Co-infections: Improvement of Neurologic Signs Including Paralysis. Three Case Reports. Abstract: 12th International Scientific Conference on Lyme Disease and other Spirochetal & Tick-borne Disorders.*

5. *Krause PJ, Spielman A, Telford SR III, et al. Persistent parasitemia after acute babesiosis. N Engl J Med. 1998;339:160-165.*

6. Shoemaker RC, Hudnell HK. *Possible estuary-associated syndrome: symptoms, vision, and treatment.* Environ Health Perspect. 2001;109:539-545.

7. Wilson ED. *Doctor's Manual for Wilson's Syndrome.* 3rd ed. Lady Lake, Fla: Muskeegee Medical Publishing, 1997.

8. Krause PJ, Lepore T, Sikand VK, et al. *Atovaquone and azithromycin for the treatment of babesiosis.* N Engl J Med. 2000;343:1454-1458.

9. Allred DR. *Babesiosis: Persistence in the face of adversity.* TRENDS in Parasitology. 2003Feb;19(2):51-55.

10. Craft JE, Fischer DK, Shimamoto GT, Steere AC. *Antigens of Borrelia burgdorferi recognized during Lyme disease. Appearance of a new immunoglobulin G response late in the illness.* J Clin Invest. 1986 Oct;78(4):934-939.

11. Logigian FL, Johnson KA, Kijewski MF. *Reversible cerebral hypoperfusion in Lyme encephalopathy.* Neurology. 1997;49:1661-1670.

12. Cheng David, Yakobi-Shvlli Rami, Fernandez Jose. *Life-threatening hypotension from babesiosis hemolysis.* AJEM. doi:10.1053/ajem.2002.27153.

13. Weiss LM. *Babesiosis in humans: a treatment review.* Expert Opin Pharmacother. 2002;3:1109-1115.

14. Stricker RB, Lautin A. *The Lyme wars: time to listen.* Expert Opin Investig Drugs. 2003;12(10):1609-1614.

Beating Chronic LYME

Chapter Two

Giving the "little bugger" credit

"Healing is a matter of time, but it is sometimes a matter of opportunity."

Hippocrates

CLD is caused by many borrelia species

Another major oversight by the medical community is that *Borrelia burgdorferi* is the only bacterium that causes Lyme disease. The truth is that there are many pathogenic borrelia strains; many of which cause borreliosis (Lyme-like disease); currently I have over 90 Lyme Disease-causing strains in my test kit. The *Borrelia strains*, become a type of spirochete when they enter their viral-like phase.

Borrelia burgdorferi sensu lato is name given to the overall category. In North America there is just one genospecies variant - *Bb sensu stricto*. In Europe there are three categories Bb sensu stricto, *B. garinii*, and *B. afzelii*. Asia has *B. garinii* and *B. afzelii*. Japan has *B. japonica* and *B. miyamoto*. These groups are evolving as new research discoveries occur.

If it were not difficult enough to get an accurate diagnosis, consider the following:

1. **There are more carriers of CLD than just the deer tick.** There is a tremendous misunderstanding regarding the vector (carrier) that transmits Lyme disease. First of all, the familiar tick vector called the deer tick and black-legged ticks (commonly called deer ticks) are more prevalent and wide-spread than previously reported. Secondly, more evidence supports the belief that ticks are not the only carrier able to transmit Borrelia species including other non-deer ticks and other insects (including mosquitos). Unfortunately, this critical information is not being reported by health officials to the public and medical community.

2. **CLD is more common than we think.** The true prevalence of Lyme disease is much higher than is being reported by health officials – heck, most 'health officials' still argue that it doesn't exist. It is difficult to estimate how many cases are unreported but it may be 10-15 times higher than what is currently

reported. Misdiagnosed cases go unreported even though Lyme disease is a mandatory reportable disease in most states.

3. **Patients need longer and more comprehensive treatment.** The standard therapy of 4 -6 weeks of antibiotic treatment is ONLY sufficient to treat ACUTE Lyme disease. Chronic Lyme disease is often a life-long illness that is then just successfully managed (that's what this book is about).

4. **Wrong diagnosis leads to wrong treatment.** I have NEVER been a fan of obtaining a 'diagnosis' as most are simply a physician's cop-out to name a set of symptoms that the patient is left to suffer with. In this case, CLD is the answer – as long as it can point the patient to the correct treatment parameters.

Reported Lyme Disease, WI,1990-2010
(n=21,704)

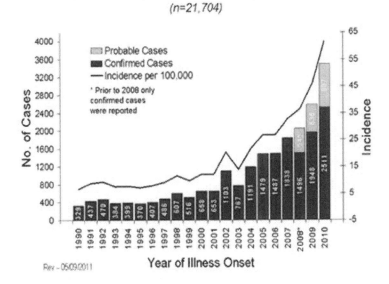

5. Lyme disease is usually accompanied by one or more co-infection:

Co-infections	Vector	Causative Agent	Endemic Area	Symptoms
Lyme Disease	Deer Tick Pacific Black-legged Tick	*Borrelia burgdorferi* *Borrelia lonsestari*	Northeast Midwest West Coast	Off season flu Rash (bull's-eye or other) Constitutional symptoms Musculoskeletal symptoms Wide range of neurological symptoms, including Bell's Palsy
Babesiosis	Deer Tick Pacific Black-legged Tick	*Babesia microti* *WA-1*	Northeast West Coast	Fever Hemolytic anemia Constitutional symptoms Possible death
Ehrlichiosis	Deer Tick Pacific Black-legged tick American Dog Tick Long Star Tick	*Ehrlichia phagocytohphila*	Northeast Upper Midwest	Fever Headache Constitutional symptoms Possible death
Colorado	Rocky	*Colorado*	Western	Fever with

Tick Fever	Mountain Wood Tick	*Tick Fever Virus*	US	remission Second bout of fever
Tick Relapsing Fever	Relapsing fever tick (Ornithodoros turicata)	*Borrelia hermsii*	Western US	Periods of fever Petechial rashes
Q Fever	Brown Dog Tick Rocky Mountain Wood Tick Lone Star Tick	*Coxiella burnetii*	Through out US	Acute fever Chills Sweats
Powassan Viral Encephalitis	Woodchuck Tick	*Flavivirus*	Eastern and Western US	Fever Meningoencephalitis 10% fatality rate 50% Neurological sequela
Rocky Mountain Spotted Fever	American Dog Tick Rocky Mountain Wood Tick	*Rickettsia*	Through out US	Sudden fever Maculopapular rash on soles of hands and feet that spreads over the entire

				body 3%-5% fatality rate
Tick Paralysis	American Dog Tick Rocky Mountain Wood Tick Lone Star Tick	*Neurotoxin excreted from tick's salivary gland*	Through out US	Fatigue Flacid paralysis Tongue and facial paralysis Convulsions Death
Tularemi a	American Dog Tick Rocky Mountain Wood Tick Lone Star Tick		Through out US	Indolent ulcers Swollen lymph nodes Deaths can occur
Bartonell a	Cats Ticks Fleas	*Bartonella Quintana Bartonella henselea*	Worldwi de	Fever Mild neurological signs Granulomatous lymphadenitis Red popular lesion

My Kinesiology test kit contains:

Anaplasma Phagocytophilum / Ehrlichia Phagocytophilum
Causes human granulocytic anaplasmosis. Symptoms may include fever,
severe headache, muscle aches (myalgia), chills and shaking, similar to
the symptoms of influenza. GI symptoms occur in less than half of
patients and a skin rash is seen in less than 10% of patients. It is also
characterized by thrombocytopenia, leukopenia, and elevated serum
transaminase levels in the majority of infected patients.

Babesia Bigemina
North and South America, Southern Europe, Africa, Asia and Australia

Babesia Bovis
Infects cattle and occasionally humans. Eradicated from the United
States by 1943, but is still present in Mexico and much of the world's
tropics.

Babesia Canis

Babesia Cati

Babesia Divergens
Has been found in Turkey, Spain, Canary Islands, Tunisia, Austria, France
and Norway. Infections have a much higher fatality rate (42%) than with
other strains and present with the most severe symptoms:
haemoglobinuria followed by jaundice, a persistently high fever, chills
and sweats. If left untreated, can develop into shock-like symptoms
with pulmonary oedema and renal failure.

Babesia Duncani
Can infect humans.

Babesia Felis

Babesia Gibsoni

Babesia Herpailuri

Babesia Jakimoni

Babesia Major

Babesia Microti / Theileria Microti
Common in US. For 25% of cases in adults and half of cases in children, the disease is asymptomatic or mild with flu-like symptoms. Symptoms are characterized by irregular fevers, chills, headaches, general lethargy, pain and malaise.

Babesia Ovate

Babesia Pantherae

Bartonella Alsaticca

Bartonella Arupensis

Bartonella Bacilliformis
Causes Carrion's disease (Oroya fever, Verruga peruana).

Bartonella Berkhoffii
Becoming more important particularly for immuno-compromised individuals.

Bartonella Birtlesii

Bartonella Bovis

Bartonella Capreoli

Bartonella Clarridgeiae
Found in domestic cats and can give humans Cat Scratch Disease

Bartonella Doshiae
May cause Cat Scratch Disease.

Bartonella Elizabethae / Rochalimaea Elizabethae
Endocarditis. Particularly among homeless IV drug users.

Bartonella Grahamii
Endocarditis and Neuroretinitis

Bartonella Henselae / Rochalimaea Henselae
Can cause bacteremia, endocarditis, bacillary angiomatosis, and peliosis
hepatis. Causes cat-scratch disease.

Bartonella Koehlerae
Human infection may be from infected cats.

Bartonella Melophagi
Discovered in 2007 and known to infect humans.

Bartonella Muris

Bartonella Peromyscus

Bartonella Quintana / Rochalimaea Quintana / Rickettsia Quintana
Causes trench fever. Can start out as an acute onset of a febrile episode,
relapsing febrile episodes, or as a persistent typhoidal illness.
Commonly seen are maculopapular rashes, conjunctivitis, headache
and myalgias, with splenomegaly being less common. Most patients
present with pain in the lower legs (shins), sore muscles of the legs and
back, and hyperaesthesia of the shins.

Bartonella Rochalimae
Carrion's disease-like symptoms.

Bartonella Schoenbuchii

Bartonella Talpae

Bartonella Taylorii

Bartonella Tribocorum

Bartonella Vinsonii / Rochalimaea vinsonii
On increase. Causes endocarditis, arthralgia, myalgia, headaches and fatigue.

Bartonella Washoensis
May cause fever and myocarditis.

Borrelia Afzelii
Has been found in Europe, USA, Singapore, Australia and New Zealand.

Borrelia Berbera
Found in Algeria, Tunisia and Libyia.

Borrelia Burgdorferi
Found in USA, Europe, Australia, New Zealand

Borrelia Carteri
Uncommon but has been found in humans in India.

Borrelia Caucasica
Found in Europe and Asia.

Borrelia Duttonii
Found in Europe and Africa. Causes Central African relapsing fever.

Borrelia Garinii
Has been found in Europe.

Borrelia Hermsii
Associated with relapsing fever. The primary cause of tick-borne relapsing fever in North America. Also found in Europe.

Borrelia Hispanica
Found in Spain, Portugal, Morocco and central Africa.

Borrelia Kochis

Borrelia Miyamotoi
Symptoms of relapsing fever. Found in Russia, Japan, Europe and North America.

Borrelia Morganii

Borrelia Novyi
Found in the Americas.

Borrelia Parkeri
Human infection.

Borrelia Persica
Found in Europe and Asia.

Borrelia Recurrentis
Found in England, Ireland, USA, Canada, Mexico, Central and South America, central Asia, Africa, and around the Mediterranean.

Borrelia Tillae
Found in Europe.

Borrelia Turicatae
Found in Europe.

Borrelia Valaisiana
Causes Lyme's disease.

Borrelia Venezuelensis
Causes relapsing fever in central and south America.

Borrelia Vincentii
Exists normally in the human mouth in low concentrations and safe proportions. Causes severe ulcerating gingivitis (trench mouth); typically found in those with poor oral hygiene but can also occur as a result of stress, cigarette smoking and poor nutrition; also can be found in those with serious illnesses.

Ehrlichia Chaffeensis / Human Monocytic Ehrlichiosis
Causative agent of human monocytic ehrlichiosis.

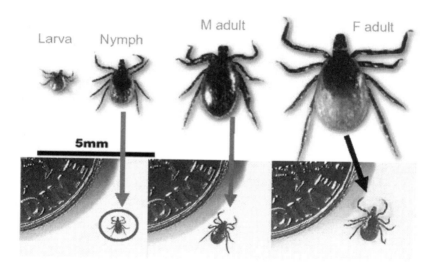

The History of Lyme Disease

According to Adams medical Encyclopedia: "Lyme disease was first reported in the United States in the town of Old Lyme, Connecticut, in 1975. In the United States, most Lyme disease infections occur in the following areas:

- Northeastern states, from Virginia to Maine

- North-central states, mostly in Wisconsin and Minnesota

- West Coast, particularly northern California

There are 3 stages of Lyme disease. (See below for symptoms.)

- Stage 1 is called early localized, acute Lyme disease. The infection is not yet widespread throughout the body.

- Stage 2 is called early disseminated Lyme disease. The bacteria have begun to spread throughout the body.

- Stage 3 is called late disseminated, chronic Lyme disease (CLD). The bacteria have spread throughout the body.

Risk factors for Lyme disease include:

- Doing outside activities that increase tick exposure (for example, gardening, hunting, or hiking) in an area where Lyme disease is known to occur

- Having a pet that may carry ticks home

- Walking in high grasses

Important facts about tick bites and Lyme disease:

- In most cases, a tick must be attached to your body for 24 - 36 hours to spread the bacteria to your blood.

- Blacklegged ticks can be so small that they are almost impossible to see. Many people with Lyme disease never even saw a tick on their body.

- Most people who are bitten by a tick do not get Lyme disease."

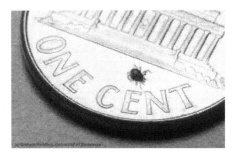

Understanding the Blood-Brain Barrier

The blood-brain-barrier (BBB) is a feature of our anatomy and physiology. There are specialized cells in our bodies that act as a blocking wall or filter, which prevents many substances from getting into our brains and spinal cord. The blood-brain-barrier makes it impossible, or at least very tough for medications to reach the brain (which is mostly a good thing—we don't want chemicals in our brains!). Throughout our bodies, we have capillaries (our smallest blood vessels), which have a lining of specialized cells (endothelial). These endothelial cells are tightly fitted together to form a filter, which protects the brain by preventing large molecules from passing through to it. Your blood-brain-barrier can be weakened by various illnesses, radiation, infection, and trauma. (4)

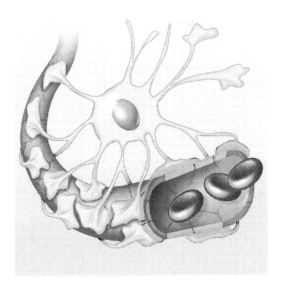

The blood–brain barrier (BBB), which is formed by the endothelial cells that line cerebral microvessels and specialized glial (brain) cells called astrocytes, have an important role in maintaining a precisely regulated microenvironment for reliable neuronal signaling in the brain. This means that when an organism like Lyme, infiltrates the brain by passing through a damaged blood-brain barrier, all sorts of bad things can happen. Most assuredly, the patient will have a local (in the brain) inflammatory process that, depending on the precise location, will alter normal neuronal conduction and mimic gross lesions. Long-term inflammation is at cause of gross lesions that then are commonly diagnosed as the disorder displayed. (1)

For example, at present there are approximately 2.1 million people that have a diagnosis of Multiple Sclerosis in America. Symptoms of MS are unpredictable; vary from person to person, and from time to time in the same person. For example: One person may experience abnormal fatigue and episodes of numbness and tingling. Another could have loss of balance and muscle coordination making walking difficult. Still another could have slurred speech, tremors, stiffness, and bladder problems.

Sometimes major symptoms disappear completely, and the person regains lost functions. In severe MS, people have symptoms on a permanent basis including partial or complete paralysis, and difficulties with vision, cognition, speech, and elimination. (2)

Just like many of our "disease diagnoses", a diagnosis of MS tells you NOTHING of the cause! Can CLD be the cause of MS? Of course it can! Is CLD ALWAYS the cause of MS? Of course NOT!

Furthermore, brain inflammation from CLD is not dependent on the Lyme spirochete itself crossing the BBB. Inflammation elsewhere in the body is defined by the release of specialized chemicals called cytokines. There are specific cytokines that are highly inflammatory and are proven to cross the BBB.

One mechanism by which blood-borne cytokines might affect the function of the central nervous system (CNS) is by crossing the blood-brain barrier (BBB) for direct interaction with the brain. Transport systems from blood to the Central Nervous System (CNS) have been described for interleukin (IL)-1α IL-1β IL-1 receptor antagonist (IL-1ra), IL-6, and tumor necrosis factor-α (TNF-α) – all inflammatory cytokines. Blood-borne cytokines have been shown to cross the BBB to enter cerebrospinal fluid and interstitial fluid spaces of the brain and spinal cord. The amount of blood-borne cytokines entering the brain is modest but comparable to that of other water-soluble compounds, such as morphine, known to cross the BBB in sufficient amounts to affect brain function. More prolonged inflammation, as seen in chronic disorders like CLD has a greater likelihood of inflammatory cytokines entering the brain to cause damage. CNS to blood efflux of cytokines has also been shown to occur, but the mechanism of passage is unclear. Taken together, the evidence shows that passage of cytokines across the BBB occurs, providing a route by which blood-borne cytokines could potentially affect brain function. (3)

Antibiotic molecules are typically too large to cross the blood-brain-barrier. And if they do get through, it is thought that they cannot penetrate in large enough quantity to have the desire effect. This makes infections of the brain difficult to treat. Although weakening of the blood-brain-barrier may make it possible for some antibiotics to break through, it is highly questionable whether or not it is safe for them to get there!

If the patient is NOT Th1 dominant autoimmune (see chapter 4), herbal remedies such as teasel, cat's claw, or samento, may be good for Lyme. While some people have found them symptomatically helpful, their molecules cannot cross the blood-brain-barrier either and can leave the patient frustrated from their ongoing neurological symptoms.

The blood-brain-barrier is NOT a factor when it comes to homeopathic whole-body, RIFE frequency healing (see chapter 5) and some other wellness-based approaches to healing. We are not trying to get chemical agents into the brain. Maybe the best treatment approach is designed to strengthen your immune system to naturally overcome illness. Comprehensive homeopathy and RIFE are 'energy medicine', not chemical approaches. Many highly reputable medical sources concur that energy medicine is a big part of the future of health care. The truth is that it has already been widely available, but not accepted or pursued by the masses in traditional Western medicine.

If you have been on antibiotics for years, in an effort to recover from Lyme, perhaps you will want to consider this information wisely. If Lyme Borrelia bacteria, as well as Bartonella, Ehrlicia, and Babesia are living in your brain, can antibiotics likely kill them? This question does not even take into account the antibiotic resistant nature of many bacteria species.

1. *Nature Reviews Neuroscience 7, 41-53 (January 2006) | doi:10.1038/nrn1824*

Astrocyte–endothelial interactions at the blood–brain barrier
N. Joan Abbot, Lars Rönnbäck & Elisabeth Hansson
2. http://www.nationalmssociety.org/about-multiple-sclerosis/what-we-know-about-ms/faqs-about-ms/index.aspx#howmany
3. **Passage of Cytokines across the Blood-Brain Barrier**
Banks W.A..[a] · Kastin A.J.[a] · Broadwell R.D.[b]
4. **THE CELL BIOLOGY OF THE BLOOD-BRAIN BARRIER**
Annual Review of Neuroscience, Vol. 22: 11-28 (Volume publication date March 1999)DOI:
*10.1146/annurev.neuro.22.1.11 **L. L. Rubin** Ontogeny, Inc., Cambridge, Massachusetts 02138-1118;*

Neurological Symptoms and CLD

CLD patients, due to inflammation in the brain from either systemic inflammation or direct infiltration of spirochetes across the blood-brain barrier may experience a number of neurological symptoms. One report cites intermittent attacks of severe headache, mild meningismus, and a predominantly lymphocytic pleocytosis. In addition to meningitis, patients may experience subtle encephalitic signs, cranial neuritis, and facial palsy. Some may develop peripheral radiculoneuritis, plexitis, or mononeuritis multiplex. (1)

Lyme disease, caused by the tick-borne spirochete *Borrelia burgdorferi*, is associated with a wide variety of neurologic manifestations. In truth, any inflammation in the brain can cause, depending on exactly where the inflammation is, disruption in normal brain function and a vast array of symptoms. (2)

There is even information that different species of Borrelia and its co-infections may trigger different manifestations of symptoms due to their predilection to attack different types of tissues. (3) None-the-less, there are countless numbers of people walking around with diagnoses of MS to ADD, Anxiety to Depression, Fibromyalgia to whatever that really have Lyme as the causative factor!

Initially, most people think of swollen and painful joints when they think of Lyme disease, if they think of anything at all. However, when you look at the symptom list below, you can see that every part of the body can be affected. The frightening collection of neurological symptoms experienced by many Lyme-disease patients is frequently called "neuro-lyme", but in fact only represents a portion of the illness.

Head, Face, Neck

- Unexplained hair loss

- Headache, mild or severe

- Twitching of facial or other muscles

- Facial paralysis (Bell's palsy)

- Tingling of nose, cheek, or face

- Stiff or painful neck, creaks and cracks

- Jaw pain or stiffness

- Sore throat

Eyes/ Vision

- Double or blurry vision

- Increased floating spots

- Pain in eyes, or swelling around eyes

- Oversensitivity to light

- Flashing lights

- Ears/Hearing

- Decreased hearing in one or both ears

- Buzzing in ears

- Pain in ears, oversensitivity to sound

- Ringing in one or both ears

Digestive and Excretory Systems

- Diarrhea

- Constipation

- Irritable bladder (trouble starting, stopping)

- Upset stomach (nausea or pain)

Musculoskeletal System

- Any joint pain or swelling

- Stiffness of joints, back, neck

- Muscle pain or cramps

Respiratory and Circulatory Systems

- Shortness of breath, cough

- Chest pain or rib soreness

- Night sweats or unexplained chills

- Heart palpitations or extra beats

- Heart blockage

Neurological System

- Tremors or unexplained shaking

- Burning or stabbing sensations in the body

- Weakness or partial paralysis

- Pressure in the head

- Numbness in body, tingling, pinpricks

- Poor balance, dizziness, difficulty walking

- Increased motion sickness

- Lightheadedness, wooziness

Psychological Well-being

- Mood swings, irritability

- Unusual depression

- Disorientation (getting or feeling lost)

- Feeling as if you are losing your mind

- Overemotional reactions, crying easily

- Too much sleep or insomnia

- Difficulty falling or staying asleep

Mental Capacity

- Memory loss (short or long term)

- Confusion, difficulty in thinking

- Difficulty with concentration or reading

- Going to the wrong place

- Speech difficulty (slurred or slow)

- Stammering speech

- Forgetting how to perform simple tasks

Reproduction and Sexuality

- Loss of sex drive

- Sexual dysfunction

Females only:

- Unexplained menstrual pain, irregularity

- Unexplained breast pain, discharge

- Pelvic pain

General Well Being

- Unexplained weight gain or loss

- Extreme fatigue

- Swollen glands

- Unexplained fevers (high- or low-grade)

- Continual infections (sinus, kidney, eye, etc.)

- Symptoms seem to change, come and go

- Pain migrates (moves) to different body parts

- Early on, experienced a flu-like illness, after which you have not since felt well

This list was compiled by Denise Lang, author of "Coping with Lyme Disease" but is by no means conclusive.

Given the fact that Lyme spirochetes can infiltrate the central nervous system within 24 hours, the designation actually applies to many more than just those disabled by neuropathic pain, hallucinations, numbness or tingling.

Columbia University established the first research center for chronic Lyme disease in the United States through the support of Lyme Disease Association (LDA), Time for Lyme, Inc, an affiliate of LDA of many other public and private donors and foundations.

The Lyme Disease Research Studies facility at Columbia University focuses on the problem of chronic Lyme disease, including the search for better diagnostic tests and treatments, drawing upon the vast resources of the Columbia University Medical Center. For more information see Columbia University's Lyme Disease Research Center.

Dr. Fallon is Associate Professor of Clinical Psychiatry at the Columbia University College of Physicians and Surgeons and is also the Director of the Lyme Disease Research Program at the New York State Psychiatric Institute. A graduate of Harvard College, he obtained his M.D. degree from the Columbia University College of Physicians and Surgeons, as well as a Master's Degree in Public Health Epidemiology from Columbia University. He is probably the foremost authority on neurological Lyme disease.

According to Dr. Fallon, Lyme disease can be easily treated if caught early. However, sometimes people don't get symptoms for *years* after they are bitten, so they don't realize they are infected.

Dr. Fallon says it is a difficult illness to have, because doctors fight among themselves about the accuracy of a patient's diagnosis (whether or not they actually have Lyme Disease) and also about how to treat the illness. Lyme also has a fluctuating symptom pattern, so a sufferer might feel fine one day, and not be able to get out of bed the next. Doctors sometimes dismiss Lyme Disease as hypochondria, and it is often misdiagnosed as a host of other disorders, including depression. He says that common symptoms are fatigue, numbness and tingling, headaches, sleep disturbances and irritability. In addition, people can often get psychiatric symptoms, including changes in mood, problems with anxiety, and even, in rare situations, paranoia or full-blown mania. (4)

Neuropathic Pain

Neuropathic pain is a complex, chronic pain that usually is accompanied by tissue injury. However with neuroborreliosis, neuropathic pain is caused by the spirochetes infecting the central nervous system and causing inflammation in the nerve endings.

With Lyme infection, the nerve fibers themselves may be damaged, dysfunctional or injured depending upon the stage of infection. These damaged nerve fibers send incorrect signals to other pain centers. Most commonly, when there is inflammation in the brain (particularly the parietal lobes) there will be corresponding sensation in the affiliated body part.

The hallmark of Lyme pain is that it "starts and stops" or "moves around". The major difference between neuropathic pain and regular pain is the acute degree of pain. "Dull" aches or "throbbing" aches would never describe neuropathic pain.

Up to 40% of patients with Lyme disease develop neurologic involvement of either the peripheral or central nervous system. Dissemination to the CNS can occur within the first few weeks after skin infection. Like syphilis, Lyme disease may have a latency period of months to years before symptoms of late infection emerge. Early signs include meningitis, encephalitis, cranial neuritis, and radiculoneuropathies. Later, encephalomyelitis and encephalopathy may occur. A broad range of psychiatric reactions have been associated with Lyme disease, including paranoia, dementia, schizophrenia, bipolar disorder, panic attacks, major depression, anorexia nervosa, and obsessive-compulsive disorder. Depressive states among patients with late Lyme disease are fairly common, ranging across studies from 26% to 66%. The microbiology of Borrelia burgdorferi sheds light on why Lyme disease can be relapsing and remitting and why it can be refractory to normal immune surveillance and standard antibiotic regimens. (5)

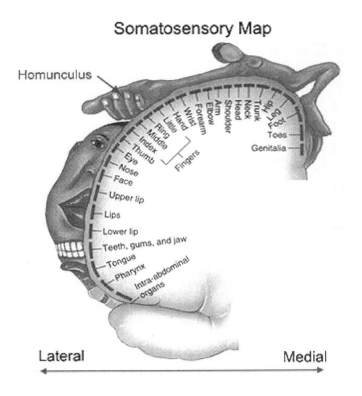

1. *The triad of neurologic manifestations of Lyme disease, Meningitis, cranial neuritis, and radiculoneuritis, Andrew R. Pachner, MD and Allen C. Steere, MD doi: 10.1212/WNL.35.1.47Neurology January 1985 vol. 35 no. 1 47*

2. *Chronic Neurologic Manifestations of Lyme Disease, Eric L. Logigian, M.D., Richard F. Kaplan, Ph.D., and Allen C. Steere, M.D. N Engl J Med 1990; 323:1438-1444November 22, 1990DOI: 10.1056/NEJM199011223232102*

3. *Different Genospecies of Borrelia burgdorferi Are Associated with Distinct Clinical Manifestations of Lyme Borreliosis, Alje P. van Dam, Herman Kuiper, Koen Vos, Anneke Widjojokusumo, Bartelt M. de Jongh, Lodewijk Spanjaard, Anton C. P. Ramselaar, Michael D. Kramer, and Jacob Dankert. From the Departments of Medical Microbiology, Neurology, and Dermatology, University of Amsterdam, Amsterdam, the Netherlands; and the Institute for Immunology, University of Heidelberg, Heidelberg, Germany Reprints or correspondence: Dr. A. P. van Dam, Department of Medical Microbiology, University of Amsterdam, AMC, Meibergdreef 15, 1105 AZ Amsterdam, the Netherlands.*

4. *http://www.neuro-lyme.com/Neuropathic_Pain.html*

5. *Lyme Disease: A Neuropsychiatric Illness, By Brian A. Fallon, M.D., M.P.H., and Jenifer A. Nields, M.D., Am J Psychiatry 151:11, November 1994 pp.1571-1580*

So How DO you Test for it?

2. **Lab Testing –**
   A. What does the CDC say? - According to the
      Center of Disease Control (CDC), they
      recommend a two-step testing procedure when
      testing blood for evidence of antibodies against
      the Lyme disease bacteria. Both steps can be
      done using the same blood sample.

      "The first step uses a testing procedure called
      "EIA" (enzyme immunoassay) or rarely, an "IFA"
      (indirect immunofluorescence assay). If this
      first step is negative, no further testing of the
      specimen is recommended. If the first step is
      positive or indeterminate (sometimes called
      "equivocal"), the second step should be
      performed. The second step uses a test called
      an immunoblot test, commonly, a "Western
      blot" test. Results are considered positive only if
      the EIA/IFA and the immunoblot are both
      positive.

      The two steps of Lyme disease testing are
      designed to be done together. CDC does not
      recommend skipping the first test and just
      doing the Western blot. Doing so will increase
      the frequency of false positive results and may
      lead to misdiagnosis and improper treatment.

      New tests may be developed as alternatives to
      one or both steps of the two-step process.
      Before CDC will recommend new tests, their
      performance must be demonstrated to be equal

to or better than the results of the existing procedure, and they must be FDA approved." (From the CDC website)

I totally disagree!

If you have symptoms that lead you to believe that you *possibly* have acute Lyme, by the time the tests come back, you may already have missed the window of treatment!

Here is the CDC's approach:

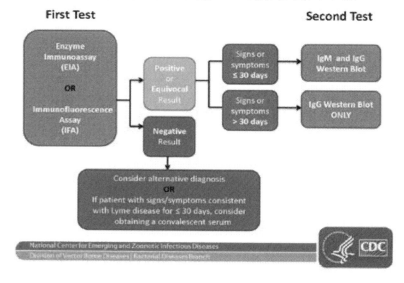

Two-Tiered Testing for Lyme Disease

First Test

Second Test

Enzyme Immunoassay (EIA)

OR

Immunofluorescence Assay (IFA)

Positive or Equivocal Result

Negative Result

Signs or symptoms ≤ 30 days → IgM and IgG Western Blot

Signs or symptoms > 30 days → IgG Western Blot ONLY

Consider alternative diagnosis
OR
If patient with signs/symptoms consistent with Lyme disease for ≤ 30 days, consider obtaining a convalescent serum

National Center for Emerging and Zoonotic Infectious Diseases
Division of Vector-Borne Diseases | Bacterial Diseases Branch

CDC

Here's REAL life:

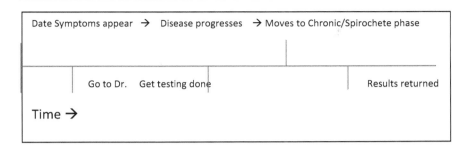

Even IF the tests performed were optimally accurate – the results usually are returned AFTER the window of opportunity pass to treat the disease with something as simple as antibiotics!

This "window of opportunity" is different in length with everyone! I've seen acute Lyme progress to chronic Lyme in a matter of days; others may be lucky enough to have weeks. This fact forces me to respectfully decline the CDC's above protocol and I think it would be prudent for you to follow suit.

B.   Other Lab Tests (most appropriate for CLD) -

IgenX Lab (see www.IgenX.com) – offers the following tests
according to their information:

The **Lyme IFA (performed as part of a Lyme Panel) detects IgG, IgM and IgA antibodies against B. burgdorferi.** IgM-
specific titers usually persist in the presence of disease. Antibody levels tend to
rise above background levels about 2-
3 weeks after infection and may remain elevated in case of
prolonged disease.

The **WESTERN
BLOT** tests (IgG and/or IgM) visualize the exact antibodies you are making to the Lyme bacteria. In some cases, the laboratory may be able to say that your "picture of Lyme antibodies" is consistent with early dis

ease or with persistent and/or recurrent disease. Not all patients have a antibodies at all times when tested. Antibodies are more commonly detected within the first year after infection, although reinfection may cause a significant rebirth of antibodies.   At most, only 70% of patients have antibodies early, and the presence of antibodies alone does not make a diagnosis of disease.

The LYME DOT BLOT ASSAY
(LDA) looks for the presence of pieces of the Lyme bacteria in urine. The assay specificity is better than 90%.

The **PCR (Polymerase Chain Reaction)** test, a highly specific and sensitive test detects the presence of the DNA of the Lyme bacteria. The PCR test is often the only marker that is positive in all stages of Lyme disease. The test can be performed on blood, serum, urine, CSF and miscellaneous fluids/tissues.

Unfortunately, Lyme bacteria like to "hide" in the body, therefore, PCR can often be negative. Studies performed on different sample types suggest that performing PCR on multiple sample types improves assay sensitivity. In the Lyme Panels, PCR on whole blood is performed as a courtesy when PCR on serum is ordered. This gives the panel 80% sensitivity.

IF I DO GET TESTED, WHICH TEST IS BEST?

Lyme disease is very complicated to diagnose because:

- Lyme bacteria are not always detectable in the whole blood, even in active disease. The bacteria like to hide.
- Every patient responds differently to an infection.
- Antibodies (WHICH IS WHAT IS TESTED) may only be present for a short time.

For patients with clinical symptoms of Lyme disease who test negative

by the IFA Screen or IgG/ IgM Western Blots, the PCR on serum and whole blood, or the LDA/Multiplex PCR Panel on urine may be appropriate.

I like the IGenX testing lab and the Pharmasan Labs (www.neurorelief.com)

CD 57- NK Cells and CTYOKINE TESTING

Personally, I don't typically do cytokine testing. But for doctors unskilled in Kinesiology, there are several labs that run these tests. See the section on autoimmune connection. However, the CD-57 testing may be the best alternative test for CLD.

Understanding the CD 57 Test:

"From coast to coast, frustrations abound among patients and clinicians regarding the diagnosis of chronic Lyme disease. Misinformed health care providers in Texas and surrounding states consider the infection rare and non-endemic. They are inclined to rule out Lyme disease based on the negative result of a laboratory test that, unbeknownst to them, is highly insensitive. In the absence of a reliable laboratory test or adequate experience in the recognition of the varied and complex presentations of the illness,most clinicians are ill-equipped to diagnose chronic Lyme disease.
Many patients suffer needlessly for years, hopelessly lost in the maze of the health care system, looking for answers and enduring the skepticism of practitioners inexperienced with the disease's signs and symptoms.

What is needed is a better Lyme test or some other objective measure to persuade the practitioner to consider the diagnosis of chronic Lyme disease. Enter the CD57 test! You may have heard the term "CD57" tossed around on chat groups, or your Lyme-literate health care provider may have even explained the test to you in one of your moments of brain-fogged stupor. What is this number that sounds more like a type of Heinz steak sauce than a lab test, and what in the world does it have to do with Lyme disease?

Let's start by going back to basic high school biology. You may remember that white blood cells (a.k.a. leukocytes) are the components of blood that help the body fight infections and other diseases. White blood cells can be categorized as either granulocytes or mononuclear leukocytes. Mononuclear leukocytes are further sub-grouped into monocytes and lymphocytes.

Lymphocytes, found in the blood, tissues and lymphoid organs, attack antigens (foreign proteins) in different ways. The main lymphocyte sub-types are B-cells, T-cells and natural killer (NK) cells. B-cells make antibodies that are stimulated by infection or vaccination. T-cells and NK cells, on the other hand, are the cellular aggressors in the immune system and are our main focus in the discussion that follows.

Let's pause a moment and introduce something you probably never learned about in high school biology class: CD markers. CD, which stands for "cluster designation", is a glycoprotein molecule on the cell surface that acts as an identifying marker. Think of comparing cells as comparing people. Humans are made up of innumerable superficial identifying characteristics (such as hair color, eye color, etc.) and so are cells. Cells probably have thousands of different identifying markers, or CDs, expressed on their surfaces, but 200 or so have been recognized and named so far.

Each different marker (or CD) on a cell is named with a number, which signifies nothing more than the order in which the CD was discovered. On any given cell there are many different cluster designation markers (CDs), giving each cell its unique appearance and function but also linking certain cells by their similarities (like grouping all people with brown hair or all people with blue eyes). Cells that have a certain kind of CD present on their surface are denoted as + for that CD type (e.g., a cell with CD57 markers on its surface is CD57+).

NK cells have their own specific surface markers. The predominant marker is CD56. The percentage of CD56+ NK cells is often measured in patients with chronic diseases as a marker of immune status: the lower the CD56 level, the weaker the immune system. You may have heard Chronic Fatigue Syndrome patients talk about their CD56 counts. A smaller population of NK cells are CD57+.

A below-normal count has been associated with chronic Lyme disease by the work of Drs. Raphael Stricker and Edward Winger. No one knows for sure why CD57+ NK cells are low in Lyme disease patients, but it is important to note that many disease states that are often confused with chronic Lyme (MS, systemic lupus, rheumatoid arthritis) are not associated with low CD57+ NK counts. The good news is that for most Lyme patients the CD57+ NK level increases as treatment progresses and health is regained.

CD57 markers can also be expressed on other kinds of cells, including T-cells, so it is important to distinguish between CD57+ T-cells and CD57+ NK cells. Clinicians need to be aware that many testing laboratories claiming to perform the CD57 test are actually looking at CD57+ T-cells rather than CD57+ NK cells, which are the cells of interest in chronic Lyme disease.

In order for a testing laboratory to measure the CD57+ NK level, it first measures the percentage of lymphocytes that are CD57+ NK cells. Then an absolute count is calculated by multiplying that percentage by the patient's total lymphocyte count. The standard normal range for the absolute CD57 NK count is 60 to 360 cells per microliter of blood. This wide range was established based upon test results of hundreds of healthy patients. By these laboratory standards, a test result below 60 cells per microliter would be considered below normal and therefore associated with chronic Lyme disease. However, a recent study of my Austin patients has led me to believe that 100 cells per microliter is a more reliable threshold separating Lyme patients and healthy controls.

When Drs. Stricker and Winger discovered that CD57+ NK cells are low in chronic Lyme patients and tend to increase with patients' clinical improvement, an opportunity arose for Lyme-literate practitioners to utilize a handy tool to aid in the diagnosis of chronic Lyme disease, to follow treatment progress, and to determine treatment endpoint. Just as AIDS patients have always held great store in their CD4 T-cell count, Lyme patients now have a fairly reliable marker of the status of their illness.

It is important to remember that the CD57 result is just a number; far more important is the patient's clinical status. An old professor of mine used to say, "treat the patient, not the lab test!" There is still much we do not know about the CD57 marker and what other factors may lower or raise it. However, overall, the CD57+ NK count is a useful tool in diagnosing and treating chronic Lyme disease in most patients. As a measure of immune status, it provides an indirect measure of bacterial load and severity of illness. Furthermore, in a patient who has a negative or indeterminate Lyme test but is highly suspect for the disease, the clinician may utilize the CD57+ NK count as one more piece in the complex puzzle of a Lyme disease diagnosis."

From: EVERYTHING YOU ALWAYS WANTED TO KNOW ABOUT THE CD57 TEST, By: GINGER SAVELY, RN, FNP-C

OTHER LYME DISEASE TESTS

- IgG/IgM/IgA Screen (IFA)*
- IgG/IgM and IgM Antibody ELISA
- C6 Peptide
- IgG Western Blot and IgM Western Blot
- 31 kDa Confirmation Test*
- Lyme Dot Blot Assay (LDA)*
- Multiplex PCR for urine, whole blood, serum, CSF
- Multiplex PCR for Miscellaneous samples (ex: Skin biopsy, breast milk)*

3. **Clinical Evaluation** – I'm just old enough to remember the days when automobile repair depended greatly on the skill and experience of qualified technician. Now, with the presence of computer chips in nearly all high-tech gadgetry, a mechanic needs sophisticated diagnostic machinery to locate the cause of my car's woes. I don't think that my mechanic is 'listening to my engine' like the specialists of the past. Doctors have evolved much the same way. They no longer listen to the patient. Let's be honest, YOU may be a better diagnostician than the doctor you pay to see!

4. **Kinesiology Evaluation** – This is a skill-set that takes years to develop and is NOT recognized by the medical profession as a legal approach to diagnose anything. I think that is a good thing as I want as little to do with the standard medical approaches as possible.
I do not diagnose, do not I practice under my chiropractic license, do not practice medicine, and do not practice to the public. Under my Pastoral Medical License, I assist members in a Biblical approach to wellness. This is one reason why I write books, blogs and newsletters. I still think that we have the right to free speech in this country and that allows me to state my opinion regardless of what the pharmaceutical companies dictate. So stated, I believe that there are better, more accurate ways to come to a conclusion that one may wish to treat their symptoms as if they are struggling with CLD. Kinesiology, properly applied, is a tool that may point people in the right direction.

You may contact my office to find out more:
www.UpperRoomWellness.com

Beating Chronic LYME

Chapter Three

Understanding the Immune Response

"When wealth is lost, nothing is lost; when health is lost, something is lost; when character is lost, all is lost."

Billy Graham

Once you've missed the "window of opportunity" of killing the pathogen with an antibiotic, things turn south. Chronic Lyme disease is, after all, what this book is supposed to be about, so what does one do?

First, one must remember that CLD usually becomes an autoimmune disorder. So it is necessary to begin with an understanding of what an autoimmune disease really is.

It is important to understand that an autoimmune disease is a 'state' that the immune system is in. It is NOT a disease of an organ; and even though it is given a multitude of names depending on the tissue currently affected, it is a STATE of the immune system attacking the tissue it was meant to protect.

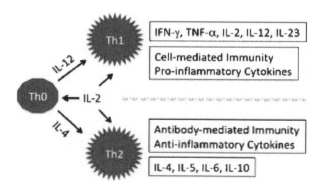

Some highlight points to know about your immune system:

- Your immune system does one thing and only one thing – it KILLS things.

- Your immune system may be separated into two responses – Th1 and Th2 (simplistically, there are more but we'll leave it at that for now)

- Your immune system is supposed to only 'turn on' against bio-toxins (living organisms like bacteria, virus, parasites...that is, things that it can kill)

- The Th1 response is the immediate, killer cell response (think of it as the Marine Corps) against the enemy and is the primary killer of antigens like Lyme pathogens and its co-infections. *What* it 'turns on' against is called an antigen in the immune response.

- The Th2 response is sent out secondarily and is mainly responsible for making antibodies against the antigen that the Th1 system 'turned on' against. The antibodies 'tag' that antigens and the Th1 system can then more easily find and kill them.

- Your immune system assists in the cleaning up of old cells necessary for cancer to NOT develop in the first place. This is primarily a Th1 function.

- Both Th1 and Th2 responses are named such because they carry a slurry of different chemicals (immune cells, chemokines and cytokines) that make up such a response.

An AUTOIMMUNE disorder happens when your immune system starts attacking self-tissue. Really, an autoimmune disease develops because your immune system has 'turned-on' against something IT FOUND lodged in self-tissue and now is destroying self-tissue as well. Let's expand that definition a little more so you can fully understand it: If my immune system fires a response against a flu virus I just picked up and it's a particularly virulent virus, a strong Th1 response is released in an attempt to kill the foreign invader and bring me back to health. My 'strong Th1 response' is really a collection of different cells that are looking for a battle; they are seeking an enemy with guns loaded. Let's say they find the flu virus and recognize that it is the enemy they were commissioned to kill, they attack it, kill it and then retreat in victory. The Th1/Th2 system goes back into balance and life is good.

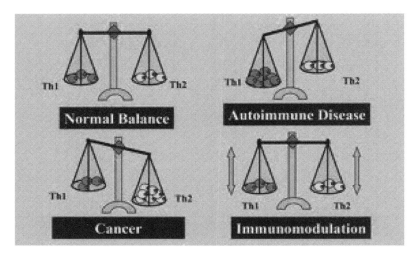

An autoimmune disease begins when, for a multitude of reasons we won't breach here, stray cytokines from a Th1 response didn't recognize the flu virus as the enemy but recognized something that they were never supposed to recognize as an enemy – let's say a heavy metal toxicity in my thyroid. Because I was exposed to a great amount of mercury from amalgams, vaccinations, and just living in a toxic world, mercury had lodge in the fat cells surrounding my thyroid and other tissues. My liver, unable to clear out that which I was exposed to, caused my system to shunt the toxicity to fat storage cells for safe keeping. Never was my immune system supposed to 'turn-on' against such chemical toxicity!

Is my immune system ever going to be able to kill mercury? Of course not; mercury is an element on the periodic table, not a living organism. If my immune system inadvertently turns-on against something that *cannot or will not die*, there will be a lot of collateral damage and I might even begin to start making antibodies against the tissues surrounding the attack. This is an autoimmune disease; it isn't really a disease at all, it is an immune attack on self-tissue because my immune system is firing against something it never should have fired against!

Remember, when the immune system turns-on against something, it does so until it achieves victory, until it kills it.

In the case of Lyme: Lyme disease in its acute state is theoretically 'killable' by one's immune system. Because it is very virulent, it may take your un-aided immune response some time to make a dent in it. This is a problem because after an indiscriminant amount of time (from a matter of a few days to several weeks), Lyme disease morphs into its spirochete (viral-like) phase and can move intracellular (within the cell).

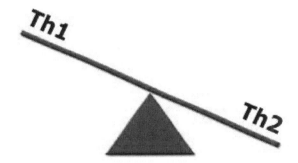

Normally, when a virus attempts to hide from one's immune response by infiltrating a cell, the cell gives off a marker on the outside of the cell membrane to alert the immune cytokines that it has been breached. Immune killer cells then engulf the entire cell, killing both the cell and the invading pathogen and protecting the whole in the process.

However, there are certain bacterial and viral organisms (Lyme being one of these) that has the capability to disarm the cell by disabling the marker that informs the immune system it has been attacked. I like to describe it this way: Think of a bank robber entering a bank and demanding the teller to fill up his bag with money. The teller pushes a secret button under the counter that summons the police and the thief is apprehended. But a smart thief (Lyme) cut the phone line outside of the building before entering the bank and the secret button does nothing to inform the police car that passes by completely unaware. Tricky little beastie isn't he?

Summary: An autoimmune disease is when one's immune system is firing against something (either predominantly Th1 dominant or predominantly Th2 dominant) that it found lodged in self-tissue that either cannot or will not die (as in Lyme) and is destroying self-tissue in the process.

So, what is the CAUSE of an autoimmune attack? It is not really an "immune system gone wrong" as it is an immune system thinking it is doing "right" but firing against something that it can never kill. The only way to ultimately correct an autoimmune disorder is to remove the antigen it is making war against. This way you are essentially fooling your immune system to think that it has won and the enemy is dead. In the case of autoimmune disease against a specific organ like Hashimoto's hypothyroidism, there is little help in direct organ support without correcting the cause. The mechanism for the issue is the immune response in the first place and not that the organ is deficient in any type of nutrient; the reason the person may need hormone replacement (such as Synthyroid) in hypothyroidism is because the immune system is actually destroying the cells, but replacement without halting the destruction is missing the point.

What does this all have to do with Lyme? Everything! Remember, Chronic Lyme (CLD) is when the acute infection has moved into a viral-like, spirochete phase that is nearly impossible to kill as it hides inside cells and evades one's immune response. When Th1 cytokines cannot find the pathogen, they start to kill surrounding tissue creating an autoimmune disorder. CLD becomes an autoimmune disorder!

Usually people with CLD that has now become an autoimmune disorder, involving much destruction and therefore many symptoms have a Th1 dominant autoimmune response, that is, the immune response is stuck in a Th1 (killer cell, Marine Corps) attack. This typically brings about much tissue damage, much inflammation and a greater number of symptoms that causes them to seek medical care and hopefully arrive at a diagnosis. They often are misdiagnosed as having MS, RA, Hashimoto's, etc. Actually, it may not be a misdiagnosis as all autoimmune disorders have an antigen at its core and that antigen might just be Lyme!

Neither the standard medical nor an alternative healthcare has adequately dealt with autoimmune conditions, including CLD, because most fail to understand the Th1/Th2 issue. Medically, the patient is given long-term antibiotics, anti-malarial drugs, steroids, anti-inflammatories and more that may temporarily relieve the symptoms but do nothing to remove the cause; alternative doctors have supported the organs with glandulars and tried to kill the CLD with herbs or other supplements. Let's face it, if either traditional medical or the alternative models had any great percentage of success treating CLD autoimmune disorder, you wouldn't be reading this book because you probably wouldn't have any symptoms.

It is important to understand that an autoimmune disease is a 'state' that the immune system is in. It is NOT a disease of an organ; and even though it is given a multitude of names depending on the tissue currently affected, it is a STATE of the immune system attacking the tissue it was meant to protect.

It's absolutely necessary to figure out if a person is Th1 or Th2 dominant because it will dictate what type of protocols that will be most effective for dampening their immune activity. We know that typical 'immune stimulants' like Astragalus, Cats Claw, Samento, Echinacea, Garlic, Glycyrrhizin, Melissa Officinalis, Maitake mushrooms, seem to stimulate the Th1 response. We also know that things like pine bark extract, grape seed extract, green tea extract, Pycnogenol, Resveratrol, and caffeine are things that stimulate the Th2 response. So if a patient's CLD attack of their joints, brain, muscles or fatigue is a Th1 dominant response, adding Th1 stimulants will MAKE THEM WORSE! You can effectively aid in balancing a Th1 dominant individual by giving Th2 stimulants and visa, versa.

It is often that the patient's history will be obvious as to which dominance they are 'stuck' in. If they've attempted taking high amounts of Cats Claw, Garlic and Echinacea in the past only to feel horribly worse afterward, there's a pretty good chance they are Th1 dominant autoimmune. If drinking green tea or coffee takes away your major symptoms, the possibility exists that you are Th1 dominant; if it made you feel worse, you may be Th2 dominant. But do NOT rely on this; it is always wise to do the testing! I wish it were always that easy to detect dominance. Many people just don't seem to get better after giving full effort with numerous nutritional or standard approaches. This should be at least a clue that there is something deeper not being addressed.

Also, you have to be very careful stimulating a Th1 or Th2 response. People can't figure out why they still feel terrible even while taking the boatload of vitamins their nutritionist recommended. If you are stimulating the dominant, hyper-firing system, you are literally throwing fuel on the fire. Autoimmune patients CANNOT take supplements that have both Th1 and Th2 stimulants. You are helping the immune system destroy your body! Do the testing!

Th1 and Th2 Balancing

There are 2 parts of your immune system, the Th1 and Th2 response. When a person is autoimmune, one of these systems is "hyper-firing" or Dominant. Balancing this system goes far in reducing a patient's symptoms:

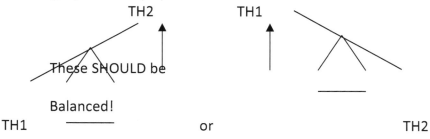

There are specific dietary changes and supplements that can help and hinder the above response: NOTE: ALL AI cases need Vitamin D, Glutathione, and Omega 3 fish oils +

Things that stimulate the Th1 response: (Take these if you are Th2 Dominant)

> Cats Claw
> Samento
> Echinacea
> Golden Seal
> Red Clover
> Pau D'Arco
> Wild Bergamot (Monarda fistulosa)
> Oregon Grape (Mahonia aquifolium)
> Andrographis (Andrographis paniculata)
> Lignan-vitae (Guaiacum officinale)
> Garlic
> Vitamin C
> Licorice root (Glycyrrhizin)
> Astragalus
> Most Medicinal mushrooms
> Most Chinese Herbs
> All "Immune Stimulants"
> Beta-glucan mushroom
> Maitake mushroom (Grifola frondosa)
> Lemon Balm (Melissa officinalis)

Things that stimulate the Th2 response: (Take these if you are Th1 Dominant)

> Caffeine (don't add this as this does a number on your adrenals)
> Green Tea
> Grape Seed Extract
> Herbal barks (Cramp Bark, Pine Bark, and White Willow Bark)
> Lycopene

Resveratrol
Pycnogenol

This is in NO way a complete list and individuals may react differently than expected!!!

Therefore, if a patient is Th1 Dominant, they should AVOID Th1 Stimulants and may TAKE Th2 Stimulants

Beating Chronic LYME

Chapter Four

Thoughts on Solutions

"I don't know the secret to success, but the secret to failure is trying to please everyone."

Bill Cosby

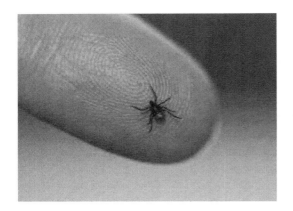

The K.I.S.S. Formula for
Acute Lyme and CLD
Phase 1 – Treating ACUTE lyme:

Initial bacterial phase – "Symptoms of early localized Lyme disease (Stage 1) begin days or weeks after infection. They are similar to the flu and may include:

- Body-wide itching

- Chills

- Fever

- General ill-feeling

- Headache

- Light-headedness or fainting

- Muscle pain

- Stiff neck

There may be a "bull's eye" rash, a flat or slightly raised red spot at the site of the tick bite. Often there is a clear area in the center. It can be quite large and expanding in size." (Adams)

Most commonly, no rash will be detected and the patient may never experience any of the above "acute phase" symptoms. This is most unfortunate as the patient is destined to move into a CLD state. If the person is bit in the head, the rash can hide under the hair and never be detected. Some people have a rash that last but a few hours; others never see a rash and mistakenly attribute their symptoms to a flu or food poisoning.

My RULE OF THUMB: If you live in a Lyme area and get flu-like symptoms during tick season, TREAT IT AS IF IT IS LYME and get an antibiotic!!! If you wait for the tests to come back, it may be too late. Find a qualified Lyme-smart MD and get a prescription.

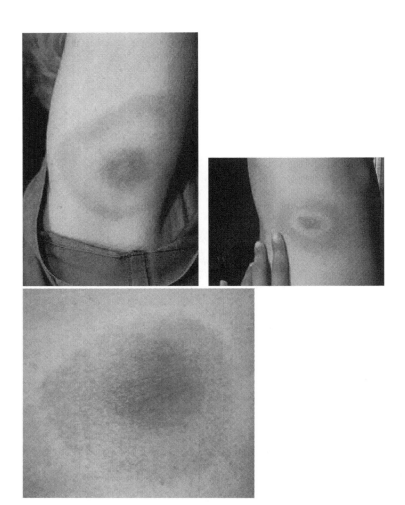

Treatment options in Phase 1:

ANTIBIOTICS

There are four types of antibiotics generally prescribed for Lyme treatment that I'd like to discuss. I am not an MD and cannot write a prescription so I'll quote Joseph J. Burrascano, M.D., *Board Member, International Lyme and Associated Diseases Society* from his 2008 work entitled "ADVANCED TOPICS IN LYME DISEASE"

1) "The TETRACYCLINES, including doxycycline and minocycline, are bacteriostatic unless given in high doses. If high blood levels are not attained, treatment failures in early and late disease are common. However, these high doses can be difficult to tolerate. For example, doxycycline can be very effective but only if adequate blood levels are achieved either by high oral doses (300 to 600 mg daily) or by parenteral administration (through an IV). Kill kinetics indicate that a large spike in blood and tissue levels is more effective than sustained levels, which is why with doxycycline, oral doses of 200 mg bid (twice per day) is more effective than 100 mg qid (four doses per day). Likewise, this is why IV doses of 400 mg once a day is more effective than any oral regimen. (I realize IV dosing is not realistic for most patients, see below)

2) PENICILLINS are bactericidal. As would be expected in managing an infection with a gram negative organism such as Bb, amoxicillin has been shown to be more effective than oral penicillin V. With cell wall agents such as the penicillins, kill kinetics indicate that sustained bactericidal levels are needed for 72 hours to be effective. Thus the goal is to try to achieve sustained blood and tissue levels. However, since blood levels are extremely variable among patients, peak and trough levels should be measured (for details, refer to the antibiotic dosage table). Because of its short half-life and need for high levels, amoxicillin is usually administered along with probenecid. An extended release formulation of amoxicillin+clavulanate ("Augmentin XR") may also be considered if adequate trough levels are difficult to attain. An attractive alternative is benzathine penicillin ("Bicillin-LA"- see below). This is an intramuscular depot injection, and although doses are relatively small, the sustained blood and tissue levels are what make this preparation so effective.

3) CEPHALOSPORINS must be of advanced generation: first generation drugs are rarely effective and second generation drugs are comparable to amoxicillin and doxycycline both in-

vitro and in-vivo. Third generation agents are currently the most effective of the cephalosporins because of their very low MBC's (0.06 for ceftriaxone), and relatively long half-life. Cephalosporins have been shown to be effective in penicillin and tetracycline failures. Cefuroxime axetil (Ceftin), a second generation agent, is also effective against staph and thus is useful in treating atypical erythema migrans that may represent a mixed infection that contains some of the more common skin pathogens in addition to Bb. Because this agent's G.I. side effects and high cost, it is not often used as first line drug. As with the penicillins, try to achieve high, sustained blood and tissue levels by frequent dosing and/or the use of probenecid. Measure peak and trough blood levels when possible. When choosing a third generation cephalosporin, there are several points to remember: Ceftriaxone is administered twice daily (an advantage for home therapy), but has 95% biliary excretion and can crystallize in the biliary tree with resultant colic and possible cholecystitis. GI excretion results in a large impact on gut flora. Biliary and superinfection problems with ceftriaxone can be lessened if this drug is given in interrupted courses (known commonly as "pulse therapy"- refer to chapter on this on page 20 of Dr. Burrascano's book for more info on this), so the current recommendation is to administer it four days in a row each week. Cefotaxime, which must be given at least every eight hours or as a continuous infusion, is less convenient, but as it has only 5% biliary excretion, it never causes biliary concretions, and may have less impact on gut flora.

4) RYTHROMYCIN has been shown to be almost ineffective as monotherapy. The azalide azithromycin is somewhat more effective but only minimally so when given orally. As an IV drug, much better results are seen. Clarithromycin is more effective as an oral agent than azithromycin, but can be difficult to tolerate due to its tendency to promote yeast overgrowth, bad aftertaste, and poor GI tolerance at the high doses needed. These problems are much less severe with the ketolide

telithromycin, which is generally well tolerated. Erythromycins (and the advanced generation derivatives mentioned above) have impressively low MBCs and they do concentrate in tissues and penetrate cells, so they theoretically should be ideal agents. So why is it that erythromycin ineffective, and why have initial clinical results with azithromycin (and to a lesser degree, clarithromycin) have been disappointing? It has been suggested that when Bb is within a cell, it is held within a vacuole and bathed in fluid of low pH, and this acidity may inactivate azithromycin and clarithromycin. Therefore, they are administered concurrently with hydroxychloroquine or amantadine, which raise vacuolar pH, rendering these antibiotics more effective. It is not known whether this same technique will make erythromycin a more effective antibiotic in LB. Another alternative is to administer azithromycin parenterally. Results are excellent, but expect to see abrupt Jarisch-Herxheimer reactions.

Real world uses:

Again, if you even THINK that you have an acute Lyme infection; antibiotics are the way to go. I do NOT suggest playing around with alternative herbs and vitamins at this stage. They tend not to kill an acute Lyme and allow the pathogen to move into the next stage.

In my two experiences with acute Lyme, I took amoxicillin with exceptional results. However, my first incidence was easy to spot with a bulls-eye rash that appeared painted upon my belly and severe flu-like symptoms. One day of 500mg amoxicillin, taken twice daily, knocked out all of my symptoms. I only completed 3 days of antibiotics though I'd never suggest anyone to follow my lead on that. The next Lyme episode went undiagnosed for nearly 5 days as I had no rash and very little exposure to the outside. At first I thought that I had food poisoning, then the flu. After 4 days I finally tested myself Kinesiologically and sure enough, it was Lyme. Amoxicillin saved the day again.

Everyone is different and for many, doxycycline is the therapy of choice for acute Lyme. It is my opinion that messing around with any other therapy to kill acute Lyme is like playing with fire. Don't do it.

Phase 2 – Treating CHRONIC Lyme

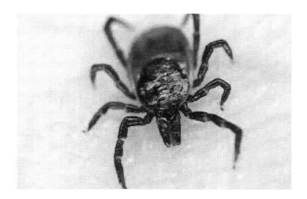

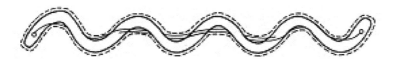

Schematic representation of a spirochete

Again, the autoimmune response is an inflammatory response, which produces chemicals called cytokines, which are part of the body's natural defense system against outside invaders. Remember, the body's immune system may be separated into a Th1 and a Th2 response. The Th1 response may be thought of as the police force or Marine Corps, the body's initial strike force against an invader or what is called an antigen.

In a PERFECT WORLD, when an antigen (this case Lyme) is present, the Th1 system fires to try to kill the Lyme; since the bug happens to be of a nasty persuasion and strong enough to resist the Th1 response, the Th2 system kicks in, creates antibodies against the Lyme, tagging them so appropriate white blood cells can finish them off. In REALITY, this rarely happens. The Th1 response is NOT strong enough to kill the Lyme pathogens and they morph into a viral-like state and go intracellular. Your Th2 cytokines start producing antibodies to the tissues it searched in and you are in for a world of trouble.

NOTE: This is a major reason WHY the blood tests for Lyme are so highly inaccurate – the quantities of antibodies are never created for a pathogen the immune system could not detect.

A person with an autoimmune disease has this process stuck in the 'on' position, either hyper-Th1 or hyper-Th2, which prolonged, destroys the tissue where the antigen is recognized. MOST CLD PATIENTS ARE TH1 DOMINANT, i.e., their immune system is 'stuck' in a Th1 phase!

Why is this so important? If the patient stuck in a Th1 dominant immune response, takes MORE Th1 stimulants, THEY GET WORSE (or at least no better). What is the main treatment modality for Lyme? Th1 stimulants!!! Um, HELLO...the patient is not going to get better!!!

Hence, if you ignore the Th1/Th2 immune response in treating a patient with CLD, both the traditional medical and the traditional alternative models of care are doomed to failure. The most important battle to fight is to calm down their immune response and stop the destruction and kill the pathogen through another route!!!

The "new model" we are proposing is simply to be more specific. If YOUR autoimmune, CLD is a hyper-Th1 attack (Th1 dominant) against Lyme and its co-infections, doesn't it make sense to do everything possible to find out how remove it while calming down the Th1 dominance? I'm no rocket scientist, but this makes sense to me. It's logical and possible to find the specific biochemical pattern perpetrating the response so we can determine how we treat them.

If you can understand this chapter and the role of the immune system, you can understand how antigens (non-living toxins or nasty, hard to kill Lyme, virus, mold, candida...) *can* be at the heart of many autoimmune disorders and even cancer.

A MAJOR part of my practice is IDENTIFYING and ELIMINATING antigens! In doing so, the body can return to homeostasis (balance) and miraculously heal itself!

Nutriceuticals

Category 1 – Things that will NOT stimulate the Th1 side of the immune response. Listed below are some nutritional approaches that will NOT mess with the immune response. By this I mean, they are usually safe for those that are Th1 dominant (which is most CLD patients):

Lauricidin (a brand name for Monolaurin that we use)

Monolaurin is in mother's milk and is a very powerful germ-fighter that is also in coconut oil. Many clinical studies have shown Monolaurin kills 100% of every pathogen (bad bacteria) it has been tested on – including the anti-biotic resistant *MRSA* staph infections! Even the FDA has approved Monolaurin for anti-bacterial food preparation. It also kills *energy draining pathogens and Lyme Disease borrelia strains!*

Monolaurin is a 12-Carbon fatty acid, derived from Coconut oil and prepared into what is called a mono-ester of lauric acid. Lauric Acid attacks viruses and bacteria by destroying the lipid coating that surrounds them which then causes their cell walls to lyse. However, it is not effective to simply take coconut oil. *Monolaurin is the mono-ester of lauric acid* which is far more biologically ACTIVE than simply the lauric acid (in pure coconut oil) at destroying viruses, bacteria, and fungi.

Pathogenic bacteria, viruses, molds and borrelia burgdorferi have a lipid fat exterior envelope or skin. This is by design so the bacteria and virus can easily move around, some even penetrating cells as described earlier. Monolaurin happens to have the same size lipid fat molecules so they *absorb into the pathogen's skin*. This can cause the lipid envelope to rupture and the bacteria or virus disintegrates and dies.

As Lyme dies, the blood then takes the debris to the liver where it is eliminated from the body. Like any of the Lyme-killers I describe, one MUST be careful about the RATE of die-off. Monolaurin is so good at what it does that it can kill bacteria and virus *faster* than then the liver can get rid of the dead cells. For this reason, I recommend that people slowly build up to a full daily treatment amount (1 tsp. of little pellets, 3 times a day) over the first week or so.

Monolaurin kills bacteria, Lyme's Disease and some viruses on *contact* with them (by absorption and disruption) and NOT by stimulating the immune response. This is why it is safe for Th1 dominant individuals. Like most things I recommend, one must remember that treating CLD is a PROCESS and takes many months or years. Taking Monolaurin over this entire time can also kill additional pathogens and Lyme bacteria when they emerge from cells they often hide in.

Colloidal Silver

Personally, I don't recommend Colloidal silver therapy for Lyme disease very often. There is some controversy regarding this therapy regarding systemic care – meaning, many think that it is not very effective past the stomach and first part of the small intestine. However, it is a great topical antiseptic and works well for stomach infections. On the positive side, one may be able to get colloidal silver into the blood and benefit from its antiseptic properties by using it in an inhaled form through a nebulizer. The size of the colloidal particles is also important. The smaller the particles size of Colloidal Silver the better the bioavailability, the stronger the anti-microbial effect and the safer to use.

MMS Protocol

MMS - Master Mineral Solution - Discovered by Archbishop Jim Humble in 1996 as an effective treatment for Malaria, has been called Master Mineral Solution, Miracle Mineral Solution and Miracle Mineral Supplement. MMS is drops of Chlorine dioxide diluted in water, MMS2 is Calcium hypochlorite in water, thus turning into Hypochlorous acid, and CDS is Chlorine dioxide gas put into water.

Chlorine dioxide is the active ingredient in MMS after it is activated by a 10% citric acid solution. The Chemical formula of chlorine dioxide is ClO2. That formula shows that there is one atom of chlorine (Cl) and 2 atoms of oxygen (O2) in a molecule of chlorine dioxide. Chlorine dioxide is a gas, and MMS is used, in most cases, as a gas dissolved in water. It can be used directly on the skin, nebulized, or taken orally (this is usually what is done). Chlorine dioxide is one of the most effective killers of pathogens such as bacteria, molds, fungus, viruses, bio-film and other disease-causing microorganisms, which includes the vast majority diseases of mankind.

Making chlorine dioxide

Chlorine dioxide is generated from sodium chlorite, which is NaClO2. Sodium chlorite has a pH of 13 which means it is highly alkaline. When citric acid or most any other acid is added, they lower that pH, causing the sodium chlorite to become unstable and thus begin to release chlorine dioxide (ClO2) from the sodium chlorite (NaClO2). Normally there is water present when the acid is added, and most of the gas will remain right in that water. The solutions that you receive when you purchase MMS come in two small bottles, one NaClO2 and one just 10% citric acid. They are then mixed together, drop for drop, in equal amounts, allowed to activate and then mixed into water.

Is MMS a bleach?

MMS (drops of chlorine dioxide mixed with water) is not bleach. Every single chemical known to man can be poisonous when taken in too large of quantities. Recently - a girl died from drinking too much water. MMS is only a few drops of Chlorine dioxide (or even just Sodium chlorite) diluted in plenty of water – it simply does not have the potential to bleach anything at all.

Many of the water utility companies in the USA are now using chlorine dioxide to purify drinking water. Chances are very high that if you believe that MMS (again, diluted Chlorine dioxide) is a bleach, then my friend you are now drinking bleach in your own home.

But remember: Anything in excess, or anything that is used in too high amount -- can be bad for anyone. I highly suggest you spend some time on the below listed website and that you read Jim Humble's book before you start MMS.

http://genesis2church.org

The Fundamentals for using MMS are these: (according to www. http://genesis2church.org)

Fundamental One:
Repeated small doses are more effective than large morning and evening doses. It has been demonstrated more than 1000 times that small doses administered often, up to once each hour, are more effective than large doses administered once or twice a day.

We now know that the chlorine dioxide chemical generated by MMS does not remain in the body more than one or two hours at most. The size of the dose does not seem to make a great deal of difference to the amount of time that MMS remains active in the body. That basically is because it doesn't matter if it is a large amount or small amount it still deteriorates into mostly just table salt in an hour or two.

So in reading the various methods of using MMS elsewhere on this web site, keep in mind - it is going to be much more effective to take MMS either each hour, or each two hours, and with smaller doses that will be equal to - or maybe larger than - one large dose.

If you are in the habit of taking larger MMS doses only in the morning and evening as was suggested in the past, MMS will still cleanse the body of microbes and pathogens. However, new research clearly reveals that a smaller-but-continuous circulation of ClO2 prevents regrouping and reproduction of pathogens, especially in situations where you are fighting a specific health issue - whether a cold or herpes or hepatitis.

After you are cleaned out a maintenance dose is still the same as always, 6 drops a day of MMS along with the citric or other acids required for activation. That's for older people and 6 drops twice a week for younger people, older people being over 60.

Fundamental Two:
Decrease the number of drops as needed if diarrhea or nausea occur, but do not stop taking MMS. Nausea and diarrhea are both good indicator signs that MMS is working. Diarrhea lasting for an hour or two is very good, but to keep it up for any amount of time can cause more harm than good. So always decrease the drops when these temporary barriers arise - they are temporary in most cases.

Fundamental Three:
Never take more than 3 drops an hour unless in a life threatening condition.

Fundamental Four:
Avoid all forms of Vitamin C for two hours before and after use of MMS. This is a temporary requirement, necessary during the significant weeks of your ramping up to the level of drops where you can be considered to be "Cleaned Out." If you are taking Vitamin C capsules marked as "12 hour" type, you will have to discontinue their use and

only take capsules or tablets that do not indicate a timed action and take them only at night after MMS hours.

Fundamental Five:
Thoughtfully maintain a nutrition program adequate to maintain your immune system. MMS takes unwanted pathogens and parasites out of your body with great efficiency but it provides no nutritional minerals or vitamins. Maintain intake of friendly micro-organisms (acidophilus and other flora). MMS itself does not kill intestinal friendly micro-organisms but forceful diarrhea can sometimes reduce their numbers. Similarly, maintain intake of minerals - especially calcium and magnesium.

Nutritional intake is critical to the immune system. Daily sunshine on the skin will maintain your vitamin D or, if you rarely see the sun, you must maintain "D" with supplements - - essential for maintaining the immune system. While MMS is the most potent germicidal agent on the planet, only the immune system produces healing and maintenance of health.

The five fundamentals above are basic to all the various methods and protocols that are explained on this Web Site: http://genesis2church.org. Be sure to click through to the various specific protocols that are highlighted below.

Six proven ways to move MMS into your body:

1. Drink it. Swallow activated MMS with any amount of water or juice flavoring added. This is the most common method. Adding water or limited juice to the mix after the three minute wait enables you to drink the mixture. The amount of water matters very little provided that you drink it all - typically one half to a full glass of water. If you drink the entire amount you will get all of the MMS benefit. Diluted little or much it will still do the same cleansing within in your body.

After the three minute wait, when you add water or juice, no more chlorine dioxide is generated. It is locked into the water or juice. After drinking the mix with the water added, the ClO2 gas will circulate in the body for less than two hours as described above. Insignificant amounts of ClO2 are generated after the water is added, but not enough to consider.

You could repeat any MMS dose every two hours (or less) without harm provided you observe the temporary barriers created by diarrhea or nausea.

2. You can spray activated MMS on skin anywhere. It is effective against localized skin sores or diseases. The mixture must have a small amount of water added to make the liquid ready for spraying. It does not bleach hair and does not harm the skin. If you have open sores or cuts, it may cause sensations of burning but it promotes rapid germ-free closure of wounds.

3. MMS retention enemas are effective in cleansing intestinal walls. They also cause the ClO2 to be absorbed and mixed with the plasma of the blood - the blood liquid. MMS benefits are more available to more parts of the body more quickly when the ClO2 is carried in the plasma.

4. Hot tub baths with activated MMS in the water expose the entire skin surface to ClO2 ions. Add hot water continually while sitting in the tub. Skin pores open and the ClO2 ions pass deep below the skin and into muscles. Since blood is always present in muscles, the ClO2 ions merge into the plasma of the blood providing greater concentration of detoxifying action against parasites, yeast, fungus and other pathogens.

5. Some people briefly breathe the ClO2 gas into the nose, head, and sinuses. <u>DO NOT DEEPLY BREATH the ClO2 gas into the lungs</u> because damage can happen to the lungs without you feeling it. Later you will find that you can almost not breathSitting with your mouth or nose over a cup of activated 2 drop mixture (definitely no more than 2 drops), and with no water added, draw the odorous ClO2 gas into the nostrils or mouth. Approach this with caution. If it seems too strong move the cup further away or prepare a weaker mixture. The first time should be no more that two small breaths until you feel a tiny "Bite."This has proven effective in killing germs in the sinuses that are often the cause of post-nasal drip. One or two brief nasal breathing session have been reported to eliminate post-nasal drip after all other medicines had failed to stop it.

Caution: If you have any history of asthma, use low doses and stop immediately if you have any sensation of an asthma attack. Never exceed the 4 drop maximum. This method is effective in situations where sinuses, vocal cords, or ear infections are retaining germs or pathogens.

Remember, it is the ClO2 Ion - the gas that you can smell - that is the germicidal agent. Use a 2 to 4 drop dose activated with 5 drops of citric acid or vinegar for each drop of MMS that you use. There's no need to add water since you won't be drinking it. Germs live and thrive in MUCUS and PHLEHM. The odor of ClO2 can kill them and prevent further production of mucus.

NOTE: Some people report "catching a cold" when using this method. Yes, there can be strong mucus films in your lungs from a cold you had a year ago known as Biofilm. Biofilm is also known in industry. Germs are sometimes encapsulated in the hardened but live mucus. The ClO2 gas weakens the mucus and the former cold germs excape. In this case, continue with internal 2 drop doses of activated MMS every hour (drink it), and continue deep breathing every four hours from the cup (Observe the limits and cautions above). The cold will soon vanish.

CAUTION: DO NOT EXCEED the 4 drop maximum mixture and take one one or two breaths. You can always mix a second dose later if you want more time span. Bird cages and free-flying house birds should be kept in another room because of their sensitivity to various gases. HEED THESE CAUTIONS. You are responsible for using this strategy responsibly so avoid prolonged deep breathing of the ClO2 gas, always separated with deep breathing of normal air.

6. DMSO can sometimes be added to the MMS activated mix in special or life-threatening situations. Special DMSO instructions are located under the 3000 protocol. Always test yourself first with a small DMSO spot on your arm. People who have a damaged or weakened liver should reduce the use of DMSO if any aching or pain is felt in the liver area. Put 1 or 2 drops of DMSO on your arm and rub it in. Wait for several hours. If there is no liver pain, you are probably safe in using DMSO.

One tablespoon of DMSO with two or more tablespoons of water can be taken internally by drinking it once or twice a day while fighting a severe disease. Normally use juice and dilute the DMSO much more. A 50-50 dilution will burn most people's throat. It's best to dilute DMSO with at least 2 parts water or juice to 1 part DMSO.

Caution One: Obviously, **DO NOT ATTEMPT any experimental intravenous injections in your home**. There are health clinics that can administer such therapies. Seek qualified professionals who can take responsibility for proper dosage, administration, and predictable outcomes from any IV process. Intravenous provides about the same benefits as methods 4 and 5 above, but at a high cost.

Caution Two: **If you choose to put activated MMS into a dehumidifier** or room fogger, keep the MMS mixture at no more than 20 activated drops per gallon of water. (Must be activated in a cup with the three minute wait before dropping it into the water tank.) People have written asking about this. They want to use the humidifier because ClO2 is a powerful deodorizer and air purifier. Remove canaries and parrots from the room.

It is best not to sleep in the room where the humidifier is fogging the room with ClO2 in the mix. Your lungs pick up the ClO2 gas (which may be beneficial) just as readily as they pick up oxygen. While the ClO2 is received willingly by your lungs and red blood cells, you could unknowingly reduce oxygen intake and suffer harm. Remember this also if children are playing or sleeping in the same room. A limited amount of

ClO2 in the air would be helpful for children and adults, but only if alert people are present and are knowledgeable about the nature of ClO2 as a germicidal agent.

It is equally effective to rid a closet or room of mold, odors, or germs if you set a 50 drop mix of activated MMS on a saucer in the middle of a closed room and let the ClO2 gas arise out of the liquid naturally. Do not add any water in this case. Do not exceed the 10 drop suggestion. It's more effective and safer to do several repeated room cleansings every hour than to release too much ClO2 at one time into a closed room. The odor does not linger and will not harm cushions, curtains, or lampshades. After 2 hours, the odor will have sacrificed itself and any room odors will be gone. If the normal small from shoes and clothes in a closet are still present, then a second ClO2 saucer or cup should be repeated.

ClO2 gas is a powerful deodorizer and germicidal agent. Drifting through the air, it will eventually kill all germs in the air and in furniture fabrics. After about two hours, the ClO2 gas disappears. It deteriorates into two molecules of water vapor. Activated MMS can restore lawn chairs thought to be ruined by skunk spray. Scrub the MMS mixture into car carpets, smelly shoes, and under arms. Will the whole house start to smell like a motel swimming pool? No, but you may expect some odor.

When using MMS as a room deodorizer or fungus eliminator, close the room doors and remove all pets and birds from the room for one or two hours.

Caution Three: **Regarding Citric Acid**: It is unusual to experience any nausea when starting MMS with a one drop dose. If you experience nausea after taking the first one-drop dose of MMS, it's rare, but you may be allergic to citric acid at the 10% solution strength. To quickly stop the nausea, wait ten minutes, then counter it with a teaspoon of baking soda in water if the nausea persists. Also eat an apple if you can keep it down. Wait overnight, then try a one-drop dose again, but use unfiltered and unpasteurized apple cider vinegar as the acid instead of citric acid.

It is very rare, but a few people are allergic to 10% citric acid in water, even though they may easily tolerate weak forms of it as in lemonade. The solution is to adopt unfiltered vinegar as the acid of choice because it is non-allergenic. Therefore try MMS again using unfiltered unpasteurized vinegar as the activating acid and slowly ramp upward in the number of drops.

Final Note: Please read the book that Jim Humble wrote to learn more about MMS!

pH Balancing and the Hydrochloric Acid Protocol

1. Alkalize Your Body. Alkaline minerals are essential for proper pH balancing and elimination of any toxic substances. They support bones, joints and whole body oxygenation. Take pH tests daily as directed in the pH Story. If you do not pass the pH tests, then follow these directions on how to replenish your mineral reserve:

   a. Eat an 80 - 100% alkaline forming diet including lots of green vegetables, drink lots of green juices like kale, celery and cucumber and use the pH Trio (Coral Legend, AloePro, D3 Serum). If you have Irritable Bowel Syndrome or digestive concerns, you may want to steam or cook your vegetables, avoid or limit the green juice and see our Intestinal Cleanse Protocol.

   b. Always avoid meat, standard animal products, soda, sugar and white flour.

c. Use GastroVen (Premier Research Labs) for 4 days before starting the rest of the program. Empty 3 Vcaps into hot water, steep for 10-15 minutes, drink 3 times per day before meals. If you have a weak stomach or interference fields (blockages in acupuncture meridian pathways – usually determined through Applied Kinesiology or QRA testing) possibly reflexing to the stomach (see below), then continue with GastroVen for the duration of the program. If you have no problem with digestion or with any of the supplements, especially the higher doses of HCL, then you can stop the GastroVen at that point.

d. Take The Following Supplements Twice Per Day: (for more information we can e-mail you details on each product listed)

- RenaVen – Superb kidney support, crucial when clearing the blood stream of waste products.

- Premier HCL – This is the main player. HCL is normally produced by your stomach for digestion and as protection against micro-organisms. But as we age, we don't produce enough. The HCL promotes adequate stomach digestion and strips the outer layer off the spirochetes. Start with one capsule after each meal. In the Strengthening Phase (first month or two), gradually build up to 2-6 immediately after meals (6-18 capsules per day).

- Once your pH is balanced and you are comfortable with the higher amounts of HCL, then continue increasing each day until you are taking 25-30 capsules after each meal (75-90 per day). If you don't eat meat or can avoid it during the program, then 25 per meal are adequate. If you eat meat, then 30 capsules per meal are necessary.

- HCL Activator – 6 capsules per day. Take 2 immediately after meals. During the 21-day Detox phase, this product is optional, if you need to take fewer capsules or save money.

- Premier Greens or another powdered greens product – Supports broad spectrum strengthening and DNA repair. Greens provide a consistent supplementation of every nutrient necessary for optimal health, including broad-spectrum, "beyond organic" vitamins, minerals, antioxidants, enzymes, immune boosters and other phytonutrients. 2 tsp per day or more.

- Premier DHA (capsules) or Nordic Natural EPA/DHA blend– Helps restore and maintain essential fatty acid balance. Take 4 capsules daily.

e. Do the following Mud Pack/Foot Bath Procedure:

- This entire procedure will be done once - not necessary to continue every month.

- Mud Packs – see instruction sheet for Medi-Body Pack below - MagmaPacks applied externally to draw out deeply embedded toxins, including heavy metals (mercury), dioxin, petrochemicals, aniline residues (from injected anesthetics) and more, including wholesale toxin release: can eliminate up to 50% of the local bio-accumulation of toxic elements in a single application. You will do 2 or 3 packs per day (less if you are weak), one at a time and follow them with a foot soak (Medi-Bath), until you have applied 2 mud packs on each of the following 6 areas, in the order listed. Skip at least one day between days you do the packs, just get to them all twice.

- Feet – can alternate each foot, pack one at a time (doing both feet in one day).

- Hands – same instructions as feet.

- Kidneys – same instructions as feet.

- Liver

- Left & Right Intestines (Colon) – same as feet.

- Any interference fields (old scars, surgeries, broken bones, tatoos, traumas) on the torso (from the chin to pubic bone). Do them one at a time until you've packed each at least two or three times.

Once on the full program, make sure you are having regular bowel movements. If experiencing constipation, you can add the following products:

- Premier Cleanse – To help clear out pockets of waste in the intestines, which are breeding grounds for parasites. Gentle but thorough intestinal cleansing that helps body eliminate constipation. Comes in powder or capsules. Take 2 capsules per meal or 1 tsp. of powder in juice or water 20 minutes before eating, twice per day.

- Galactan - Great-tasting, fiber-rich nutrition from arabinogalactan; promotes enhanced immunity. Galactan promotes healthy, complete bowel eliminations and gastrointestinal health and supports beneficial GI micro flora. Take 2 tbs. daily in liquid or food.

- Noni – Supports normal bowel function when nothing else seems to help (especially in severe constipation), helps rejuvenate large and small intestines, also provides thyroid and mood support. 10 – 20 capsules per meal until unassisted bowel movement, then decrease by 3 every 3 days (as long as still having unassisted movement).Also, be sure to consume the 5 Elements

For Proper Bowel Elimination:

- Water – ½ body weight in ounces every day, less if eating primarily fruits and vegetables.

- Salt – use our Pink Salt, which is not processed, heated or demineralized table salt (even most sea salt is processed). You can also do our Pink Salt Flush.

- Probiotics – use our Kefir (very inexpensive) or miso (best brand is Yamabuki plain, not dark variety). If prior antibiotic use, then use our 12-strain Probiotic Caps for 1-2 months - Certified as 6.25 times stronger than any other lactic acid bacteria, fully "live" raw nutrient concentrate, not freeze-dried. 2-4 capsules per day, 20 minutes prior to breakfast.

- Bulking agents – eat fiber foods in your diet and/or use our Premier Cleanse or Galactan above.

- Essential Fats – use our Premier DHAs and avoid all cooked (except Coconut Oil), partially hydrogenated or fractionated oils.

Pink Salt and Vitamin C Protocol

What if two common household items--Salt and Vitamin C—could be combined into one powerfully effective way to combat the root cause of Lyme disease? Well, that'd be great.

Though no *one* thing in this book will be a cure-all for everyone, these two common items, used properly, can be a help to those with CLD. I must say that if you have high blood pressure, do NOT try this protocol!

Americans eat the WRONG type of salt! We do consume massive amounts of sodium chloride in everything, usually heavily processed foods. Many studies demonstrate that a whole host of new illnesses could be a result of our increased use of poor forms of salt and lowered consumption of mineral-rich salt. It is thought that early man consumed as much as 10-20 grams of mineral-rich salt each day. Now it is nearly impossible to buy produce (even organically grown) that has the necessary minerals and salt content. Medical researchers are now wondering if the decrease in mineral-rich salt consumption has allowed these new illnesses, such as Lyme, Chronic Fatigue Syndrome, Fibromyalgia, Alzheimer's disease, and Gulf War Syndrome to flourish.

More recently, the salt scare of the past couple of decades has been brought into question with many researchers admitting they were wrong. Don't get me wrong, consuming more that 1500-2000mg of table salt (maximum recommended by the American Heart Association) is unhealthy. I'd even go a step further to say that ANY processed table salt is unhealthy. We could even stretch that to most sea-salt brands available in the grocery stores as these are equally processed and void of both nutritional minerals and energetic properties. In addition, the U.S. Recommended Daily Allowance of Vitamin C is a mere 60 milligrams per day. Researchers like Linus Pauling are suggesting 18,000 milligrams per day would result in profound benefits for preventive health.

Taking these two common items together results in the systematic eradication of the bacteria associated with Lyme disease. But, it's even more effective than that. Recent research is showing the possibility of other pathogens being associated with Lyme disease. These pathogens may cause many of the lingering and seemingly untreatable symptoms of the disease that plague so many Lyme disease sufferers long after treatment. Additional forms of bacteria, mites, and worms all can exacerbate the typical symptoms and presentation of the disease. The "72 Hour Remedy" acts to wipe out these largely hidden causes of the disease quickly, painlessly, and with unbelievable effectiveness.

Dosage

- 12 capsules of pink salt per day (1/hour). The only brand I have used and would recommend is from Premier Research Labs (PRL) – you'll need to capsulize the Pink salt yourself
- 36 capsules of whole-food Premier (PRL) Vitamin C (3/hour) per day
- Water

The treatment requires that you take 1 capsule of Pink Salt and 3 capsules of Premier C every hour throughout the day with ample amounts of water, a demanding schedule but the results are well worth the slight inconvenience. Taking each dosage with food is advised to help in absorption and to reduce side effects.

The effects are sometimes immediate and powerful if the infection is of long duration and the bacteria has had a chance to establish a strong foothold in your system, however, some people just cannot tolerate starting at such doses!

It may be a better approach is to "scale up", gradually increasing the dosage and "working with" the Herxheimer reactions as they occur with the protocol. A gradual-dosage protocol, even at the initial lower quantities, can have a notable effect depending upon bacterial load, body weight, etc. In fact, a smaller person often does not have to use the entire 12 doses per day of salt and Vitamin C; 6 to 8 doses often is enough for a full effect.

In any case, indications that the body is 'flushing' toxins and attendant phenomena referred to as 'Herxheimer' reactions should suggest that the current dosage level in a gradual-dose protocol should be maintained. Once the body becomes acclimated to that level of dosage, the next higher level can be attempted. Should the Herxheimer reaction be especially arduous, return to the lower dosage until the reaction passes, then resume a gradual increase once again.

An example of a gradual-dose protocol would begin with a dose of 1 dose each of salt and Vitamin C at 10 am and again at 2 PM. If you experience fatigue or have a mild feeling of malaise, omit a 6 PM dose. Instead, drink plenty of water through the rest of the day and evening. Maintain a schedule of just 2 doses per day until there is no reaction-- this may take 1 or 2 days--then move on to 3 doses per day with the addition of a dose at 6 PM.

Continue a gradual increase until reaching the 8 -12 doses of both salt and Vitamin C. Though 12 doses a day is what the protocol asks for, there is usually a notable effect after reaching 8 doses per day. Higher doses have an increased effect where there is a "stubborn" area in the body. Once you've attained the prescribed dosage, you will begin noticing immediate results. "Bad" bacteria will begin dying almost immediately as the potent combination of Vitamin C and salt helps cleanse the body of toxins and "supercharges" the body's defenses.

Remember to drink large quantities of water--no less than 12-8 ounce glasses. This will not only serve to keep you hydrated as your body flushes itself, but also help to make sure the remedy is delivered throughout the body as needed.

If after 72 hours you do not feel better, repeat the remedy once every 3-5 days until you notice the benefits. Additional remedies are presented below to assist your body in its healing process.

Why does this protocol work?

Our white blood cells (WBC) are important parts of our immune system. Some of them display unique "mechanisms" with which they attack and kill bad bugs in our bodies, like the Borrelia b. bacteria that cause Lyme disease. One class of white blood cells in particular has areas where they store an enzyme that uses an acid, along with hydrogen peroxide, to produce an oxygen particle (electron) that kills invading microbes. In other words, it creates and uses a free radical molecule to protect itself.

Another area of storage in these same white blood cells contains different types of proteins (polypeptides), one of which is called cathelicidin. A segment of this protein is a potential bacteria killer (bacteriacide) that increases the "permeability" of the bacteria's cell membrane which ultimately kills them.

One enzyme, called "elastase" a series of short protein peptides, are able to be assembled into larger ones (dubbed "LL-37") that are able to increase the "permeability" of the bacteria's cell membrane.

These two enzymes work together when they meet an offending bacterium. The elastase uses some of the cathelicidins to pull out a protein molecule from the surface membrane of bacteria. This causes an opening or "pore" to form in the membrane itself. This allows vital potassium ions needed by the microorganism to escape from within its internal walls (the Borrelia's "cytoplasm") and out through the "pore". This damages the bacteria internally; resulting in swelling and eventually ruptures the microorganism.

Increasing the salt in the body fluids surrounding the Borrelia bacteria contributes to the killing effect by allowing sodium ions to enter the bacteria through the "pore" created by the anti-microbial peptides. The increased level of sodium in the bacteria, combined with the loss of needed potassium, enhances the killing effect further.

Vitamin C is known to increase the number and activity of white blood cells. People infected with Lyme disease often have lower white blood cell counts due to the ongoing infection. So, in addition to the known anti-microbial "osmotic pressure effect" of salt, it appears the Vitamin C may increase the number and activity of the white blood cells needed, and then the increased salt levels in the intra cellular fluid "arms" them with Borrelia-killing enzymes and peptides.

Common Side Effects

This protocol may take longer for some individuals due to the length of time the bacteria has had to create pockets of infection. However, many people with mild cases have complete remission of symptoms after even 1 or 2 days. Others have to use the protocol longer or periodically over time. As encouraging as that may be, it's important to be aware that the protocol may cause side effects in some individuals.

Because you are actively helping your body fight the bacteria, diarrhea is common. This is a sign that your body is beginning to flush out the toxins and begin renewal. This may also be a sign that your bowel has reached its tolerance for Vitamin C.

This is one of the indications of a Herxheimer reaction and also signals that healing is starting. It is widely recognized that the Herxheimer reaction is caused by the release of toxic chemicals called endotoxins released from the cell walls of dying bacteria due to effective treatment. Dorland's Medical Dictionary adds that the condition is a short-term immunological reaction which causes fever, chills, muscle pain, headaches, and skin lesions. This, in turn, results in a response from the immune system which manifests the symptoms experienced by the individual being treated.

The generalized symptoms of a Herxheimer reaction, as listed above, are not all-inclusive. The severity of the reaction is proportional to the dosage of the drug or treatment causing the reaction and a wide variety of symptoms can result if the waste products reach any specific areas of the body. In such cases, the added symptoms are localized to the area or affected system. Nausea, diarrhea and soreness of the throat may also result.

Supplementation Considerations

It is very important that one does not incorporate any nutritional supplementation program until they are tested on several fronts. First, as stated previously, inflammation from an autoimmune disorder may be either a Th1 or Th2 dominant process – they are treated VERY differently. In our office, one of the first things we do is to take patients off all their supplements. They typically enter with a bag full of vitamins, minerals and magic potions that they heard would be the cure for their ailment. They are disappointed, discouraged and have spent a small fortune 'guessing' at what might work. I can't blame them, they've been to multiple doctors and most have begun in-depth investigations for themselves, searching for anything that would bring them relief.

I hesitate giving a list of any nutrition in this book since I know that most reading it will, once again, 'try' to do this on their own. This is not meant to be a self-help book or a cookbook for brain problems. I desire that you seek care from a qualified doctor trained in Carrick Neurology, Applied Kinesiology and Functional Medicine. Sometimes a little knowledge can be dangerous; you want to do this correctly. So, I will give you guidelines, not a template. In our office we test patients on everything with blood work, urine, saliva, and Kinesiology so we don't 'waste' the patient's money with useless supplements or waste time with things that won't work. Understand, just because I list the below supplements in certain categories depending on the cause of inflammation, I do not practice cookbook nutrition and this book does not advocate it. Seek a professional's help!

Th1 Dominant CLD

A Th1 dominant autoimmune disorder and a Th1 dominant acute infection are also treated differently. An acute infection will be a Th1 response and the Th1 response should be supported nutritionally – meaning you would take Th1 stimulants to aid the body's attempt to kill a pathogen. There are some variations, so let me give you a few examples:

If I get a nasty cold or flu, I want to support my immune system with Th1 stimulants. If I step off of a curb and sprain my ankle, my body responds with a prophylactic Th1 response to kill any secondary infection and heal the site of injury, my ankle swells because of it and I may even have a fever. In this case, the Th1 response is less than necessary, assuming I didn't break my skin barrier and had no exposure to an antigen. Taking Th1 stimulants may be inappropriate and cause further inflammation; ice, a physical anti-inflammatory would be the best choice. Even a chronic problem like Lyme disease that has now turned into a Th1 autoimmune disorder may be treated with Th1 stimulants during the proliferation phases. It gets a bit complicated with Th1 dominant autoimmune diseases that are driven by a bio-toxin.

In general, patients with Th1 dominant autoimmune disorders should not be taking Th1 stimulants. Understand also that just because I list something in one category or another, every patient is different and their particular body type may react in opposite ways. No approach or expensive research study will be perfect for YOU. You are a unique individual; that is why I rely on appropriate testing. Below is a list of common Th1 stimulants that I test for in patients that are Th2 dominant, have an acute Th1 infection, or may be Th1 dominant autoimmune with a bio-toxin as the antigen and it is in its multiplication/proliferation phase:

Typical Th1 stimulants:

Vitamin C – Let's clarify some nutritional principles first: Vitamins are not individual molecular compounds, they are biological complexes. The beneficial activity of vitamins only takes place when all conditions are met within the environment, and when all co-factors and components of the entire vitamin complex (found in nature) are present and working together.

Vitamins cannot be synthesized and/or isolated from their complexes and still perform their specific life functions within our body.   Royal Lee, a genius in his time, wrote:

A vitamin is: "... a working process consisting of the nutrient, enzymes, coenzymes, antioxidants, and trace minerals activators."

> - Royal Lee "What Is a Vitamin?" Applied Trophology, Aug. 1956

Legally, vitamin C is ascorbic acid, because when it was discovered, that was all that was seen in the microscope of the day. Reality is different. Ascorbic acid is an isolate, a fraction, a distillate of naturally occurring, whole form vitamin C.   In addition to ascorbic acid, vitamin C must include rutin, bioflavonoids, Factor K, Factor J, Factor P, Tyrosinase, Ascorbinogen, and other components that it is found with in nature.

If any of these parts are missing, as in the vitamin C capsules you most commonly purchase, little to no real vitamin activity takes place in your body. When some of them are present, the body will draw on its own stores to make up the differences, so that the whole vitamin may be present. Ascorbic acid is described merely as the "antioxidant wrapper" portion of vitamin C; ascorbic acid protects the functional parts of the vitamin from rapid oxidation or breakdown. (Somer p 58 "Vitamin C: A Lesson in Keeping An Open Mind" The Nutrition Report)

Most of the ascorbic acid in this country is manufactured at a facility in Nutley, New Jersey, owned by Hoffman-LaRoche, one of the world's biggest drug manufacturers where ascorbic acid is made from a process involving cornstarch and volatile acids. Most vitamin companies buy the bulk ascorbic acid from this single facility and create their own labels, combinations, claims, formulations, and unique 'twists' to claim to have the superior form of vitamin C, even though it all came from the same place, and it's really not really vitamin C at all.

This is really the story of all the vitamins. Most are synthetic, manmade, created in a laboratory and yet legally labeled as the real vitamin. By contrast, "whole-food vitamins" are created from the entire food that contains the nutrient in abundance. They typically contain far less of the nutrient on the label but they are much more 'active' and really work in your body. Again, I'm not even saying that there is no benefit in ascorbic acid; I've seen high-dose, intravenous ascorbic acid therapy work for some cancer patients. What I am say is that ascorbic acid is NOT the whole vitamin found in nature and may NOT be the best choice in daily or therapeutic use. We use whole-food nutrients as often as possible and suggest the same.

Cat's Claw (Uncaria tomentosa, Uncaria guianensis, Una de Gato, Samento, Saventaro) is an herb traditionally used by the Asháninka Indians of Peru. The tribe recognized two different types of this plant (one was used therapeutically, the other was rarely used). This difference has been verified phytochemically and two chemotypes have been identified: the preferred chemotype contains predominantly only pentacyclic oxindole alkaloids (POAs) speciophylline, mitraphylline, pteropodine, isomitraphylline and isopteropodine; the other chemotype, which was never used, contains predominantly the tetracyclic oxindole alkaloids (TOAs) rhynchophylline and isorhynchophylline in addition to the POAs. The preference for the POA chemotype Cat's Claw has been backed up by scientific research even though there has been more than enough puff made about TOAs, we still must point out that all Cat's Claw contains some. I like to use a product that utilizes the synergistic benefits of Cat's Claw with a few other herbs. Coriolus, Green Tea and Olive Leaf extract blend well with Cat's Claw.

Cat's Claw acts as an immune stimulant, it aids the Th1 response. It also has some anti-inflammatory actions as well and is therefore a great benefit to a bio-toxin generated autoimmune disorder in the brain. Because of its anti-inflammatory benefits, it can help brain issues like depression, anxiety, ADD/ADHD and the like.

Cat's Claw is particularly beneficial in treating Lyme disease. Lyme just may be the most misdiagnosed problem in America leading to many autoimmune disorders. Doctors are inclined to rule out Lyme disease based on the negative result of a laboratory test that are just plain poor! Since there has been no reliable laboratory test for Lyme, most clinicians are ill-equipped to diagnose chronic Lyme disease and I have had scores of patients that were refused treatment of acute Lyme due to a false negative test. These are the patients who have suffered needlessly for years, hopelessly lost in the maze of the health care system, looking for answers and enduring the skepticism of practitioners inexperienced with autoimmune disease.

What has been needed for years has been a better Lyme test or some other objective measure
to persuade practitioners to consider the diagnosis of chronic Lyme disease.

Recently, researchers Dr. Raphael Stricker and Dr. Edward Winger discovered that chronic Lyme patients exhibit a decrease in a specific marker called CD57+. White blood cells (a.k.a. eukocytes) are the components of blood that help the body fight infections and other diseases. White blood cells are categorized as either granulocytes or mononuclear leukocytes. Mononuclear leukocytes are further sub-grouped into monocytes and lymphocytes.

The main lymphocyte sub-types are B-cells, T-cells and natural killer (NK) cells. B-cells (part of the Th2 response) make antibodies after the T-cells in the Th1 response fail to destroy the antigen in 'round one'. T-cells and NK cells are the initial cellular aggressors in the immune system and are the sub-group that the CD57 markers are a piece of.

CD markers are a part of the chemical slurry making up an immune response. CD, which
stands for "cluster designation", is a glycoprotein molecule on the cell surface that acts as an identifying marker. Cells have thousands of different identifying markers, or CDs, expressed on their surfaces, and about 200 or so have been recognized and named so far.

Natural Killer cells have their own specific surface markers; the predominant NK cell marker is CD56. The percentage of CD56 NK cells is often measured in patients with chronic diseases as a marker of immune status, i.e., the lower the CD56 level, the weaker that particular portion of the immune system. With chronic Lyme disease, Dr. Raphael Stricker and Dr. Edward Winger discovered, CD57 NK cells are lower than individuals that are healthy and lower than patients suffering from other chronic, autoimmune disorders. This makes measuring CD57 counts a great marker for these chronic patients who often think they are going crazy.

The reason I bore you with the details is that Cat's Claw has been shown to be a tremendous help to increase CD57 values. Who knows what other diseases may be helped with increased CD57 markers.

Artemisinin – Is the active constituent of the herb *(Artemesia annua)*. Tea made from this herb has been used in Asia to successfully treat malaria. Artemisinin (pronounced art-ee-MISS-in-in) is the preferred antimalarial therapy. It is also being used to treat cancer in veterinary medicine and is an effective anti-parasite and anti-microbial treatment. Artemisinin also seems effective in treating CLD. There are many testimonials from users claiming significant benefits.

GoCLDenseal root – The best brand out there is may be Eclectic Institute's freeze-dried goCLDenseal root. This can be another helpful product for some with CLD. Personally, I have not found that it tests out very often.

Teasel – Another effective herbal therapy that is becoming a 'hot topic' more

Olive Leaf Extract – (Oleuropein) Must be taken at high doses though. Take 1500 – 2000 mg three times per day.

Garlic – Antimicrobial and helps reduce blood clotting. Use fresh garlic or freeze-dried supplements.

European (or Hungarian) Mistletoe – There is a little information that this may be beneficial for CLD as an antimicrobial.

Typical Th2 stimulants:

Immune modulators – things that should be tested to help balance either side:

Andrographis (Andrographis paniculata, green chiretta, chua xin lian, senshinren) – Andrographis readily crosses the blood-brain barrier so it can be very effective in modulating immune responses in the brain. It is a great antispirochetal agent so can be extremely beneficial for a chronic Lyme patient. Its benefits to reduce neuro-inflammation may be one of its greatest aids, but it has been used for centuries by various cultures to treat everything from malaria to pandemic flu. It is very effective for a variety of parasitic infections and was a primary treatment for syphilis prior to antibiotic use.

I believe that the primary function of Andrographis is in down regulating iNOS (cytokine inducible nitric oxide synthase – the pro-inflammatory or 'bad' NOS that gets 'revved up' in autoimmune disorders). When iNOS increases, the 'good', anti-inflammatory, epithelial nitric oxide synthase (eNOS) gets reduced. eNOS is necessary for vessel wall health and essential to keep healthy barriers like the blood-brain barrier, gut barrier, as well as arteriole wall integrity in heart disease and strokes. This, I believe, is why Andrographis has been proven to help heal patients following heart surgery, angioplasty, and myocardial infarction. It is really one of the 'good guys' in healing the brain and other tissues.

Japanese Knotweed (Polygonum cuspidatum, Chinese knotweed, Hu Zhang, Kojo, Itadori, Hojang) – Though this can act as a Th1 stimulator and must be tested in individual patients, Japanese knotweed can work well to modulate the immune response. Studies have revealed antiparasitic, antibacterial, antifungal, anticancer properties as well as central nervous system calming properties. It also protects the body against endotoxin damage from 'die-off' of bio-toxins killed through other sources. Other studies have shown it to be anti-inflammatory and may be extremely useful in calming Th17 inflammation in the brain as it crosses the blood-brain barrier readily.

Some bio-toxins (living organisms invading the body) can release compounds called matrix metalloproteinases (MMPs, of which there are several different types) that destroy our body's tissue. Many anti-inflammatories that I highly recommend in this group have shown to help clear the body of these MMPs, but only one, Japanese knotweed, has proven to block several types of MMP production. It also contains Resveratrol, by itself a Th2 stimulant, but in combination with the whole herb, it acts to inhibit MMP levels as well. Other research has shown that it inhibits arachidonic acid metabolites that force the COX inflammatory pathways as well as iNOS (the 'bad' nitric oxide that causes inflammation in the brain). It has also been proven to interfere with nuclear factor-kappaB, a chemical linked to inflammation, autoimmune disorders and cancer. It helps regulate normal cell death (apoptosis) where that has been altered (in cancer), and just modulates the immune response, especially in the brain and spinal cord.

Knotweed has also show to increase circulation to the small vessels of the eye, ear, joints, heart and skin. I test all Lyme, Hepatitis C, and other bio-toxic patients on knotweed. It can also work well for acute infections.

Other Common Nutritional Approaches:

Cat's Claw / Samento / Saventero – A Peruvian herb *(Uncaria tomentosa)* is quickly becoming a rising star within the CLD community. It appears to have both anti-microbial and anti-inflammatory properties both of which are significantly effective. Tolerance is a question for some. It can cause anxiety, insomnia, and irritability in certain individuals. Adjusting the dose appropriately can control this side-effect. Even at very low doses it seems to be beneficial.

Enzyme Therapy

Proteolytic enzymes (also called: pancreatic enzymes) as well as other enzymes, literally cut apart the thick protein coating which covers and protects Lyme spirochetes. Proteolytic enzymes are normally used to cut apart the protein coating so that the immune system can recognize the cells as pathogens. The use of Proteolytic enzymes for this reason has been around for decades.

By cutting apart the protein coating Proteolytic enzymes may also be able to get much more of another therapy inside the cancer cells. By this I mean that typically, one would NOT use enzyme therapy ALONE. Enzymes are something you ADD to your current therapy to cut through the pathogen 'bio-film'. These are commonly used to treat cancer, candida and mold!

There are many, many brands of Proteolytic enzyme supplements. One of the best that I've found is called Interfase Plus from Klaire Labs. Build up to 1-3 pills, three times a day for the standard doses. Higher doses can be used as well but these MUST be taken on a relatively empty stomach (or they work to digest your food, which is great but NOT what we are trying to do here).

Enzymes are necessary for a healthy digestive system; the enzymes present in raw foods work synergistically with the body's endogenous enzymes to digest food components completely and effectively. However, cooking and heat processing destroy raw food enzymes, placing the full burden of digestion on the pancreas and other digestive organs. Certain health conditions can also affect the body's ability to produce its own enzymes, resulting in fewer enzymes excreted from the pancreas, stomach, and brush-border membrane of the small intestine. Both of these situations can adversely affect the gastrointestinal system as well as the rest of the body, leading to common problems such as abdominal pain, bloating, gas, indigestion, gastric reflux, constipation, diarrhea, and yes, even cancer or the endless growth of pathogens like CLD.

Over time, impaired digestion can lead to an increase in intestinal permeability, or "leaky gut." Undigested protein molecules can also cross the intestinal lining and trigger immunological reactions that can be the precursor to autoimmune disorders.

Research has shown that one way to support the digestive process is to supplement the diet with plant-, microbial-, or animal-derived enzymes. Supplemental enzymes can assist in the breakdown of food, reduce the number of large and potentially inflammatory molecules leaking through the intestinal membrane, and enhance the absorption of vitamins and minerals by reducing food to its essential elements. This is the essence of Dr. Kelley's famous "high-dose enzyme therapy" for cancer patients. We use a variety of plant/microbial-derived enzymes that are active across a very broad pH range, making them effective throughout the entire GI tract.

Populations of microorganisms in the human gut are divided between free-living planktonic microbes and colonizing sessile biofilm organisms. Biofilm consists of microorganisms encased within a self-produced matrix of exopolysaccharides and exoproteins that strongly adheres to interfaces and resists dislodgement.

Microorganisms residing within biofilms are highly resistant to antimicrobials including antibiotics and bacteriocins produced by probiotics. The biofilm of healthful commensal microorganisms greatly contributes to intestinal barrier function and colonization resistance. Disrupted healthful biofilm permits colonization and biofilm formation by potential pathogens such as Klebsiella pneumoniae, Escherichia coli, and Candida albicans. Eradication of pathogen-associated biofilm is critical to successful elimination of these harmful organisms and restoration of healthful biofilm communities. InterFase® is a highly specialized enzyme formula that supports normal gastrointestinal function and microflora by assisting degradation of biofilm communities of potentially pathogenic CLD bacteria, mold, yeast, and all co-infections.

Hydrogen Peroxide

Hydrogen Peroxide – (H2O2) Is a potent antiseptic but I'm concerned about the safety of oral and IV administration! This, like every other therapy described in this book should ONLY be used under the direction of your physician.

Controlling cancer (or any chronic disease such as CLD) can be done by controlling the oxygen and/or controlling the things that free up oxygen (e.g. ionized water) and other ways. Hydrogen peroxide, and other oxygen therapies, are one of the most widely used therapies world-wide because they provide oxygen to the sick cells. They are safe and effective if used CAREFULLY. H2O2 is also used for a host of other ailments, including AIDS and any other virus based illness.

I want to emphasize very strongly that you should not use any type of hydrogen peroxide unless it is "Food Grade." The junk you buy at grocery stores and most health food stores is high in iron and who knows what other chemicals (as a minimum they are not removed) and is for EXTERNAL USE ONLY.

There is no controversy about H2O2 being used topically (i.e. externally) or with an I.V. However, there is a major controversy about whether it should be taken orally.

- *"The most common form of hydrogen peroxide therapy used by doctors is as an intravenous drip. For use at home, some individuals add a cup of 35% food grade hydrogen peroxide [or 10 cups of 3%] to a bathtub of warm water and soak for 20 to 30 minutes as the hydrogen peroxide is absorbed through the skin. Others drink a glass of water to which several drops or more of food or reagent grade hydrogen peroxide have been added [note: use Food Grade H2O2]. Although there have been reports of improved health with oral use, physicians like Dr. Farr believed that taking hydrogen peroxide orally could have a corrosive and tumorous effect on the stomach and small intestine and advised against using it. There is animal research supporting this caution."*
http://www.diagnose-me.com/treat/T216805.html

Actually, if you added 4 cups of 35% H2O2 to the bath water it would only be about a 1/5 of 1% solution of H2O2 (assuming 45 gallons are in the tub).

Robert O. Young, PhD is another person who recommends against taking H2O2 internally. In his book "Sick and Tired?" he states:

- *"Some health practitioners have given hydrogen peroxide internally to patients. There have been some reports of success*

with this, but it is highly controversial. My opinion is that it should never be used internally for any reason. For one thing, it is not a nutrient, and the risk of it combining in the body with superoxide is too great."
"Sick and Tired?", page 74.

His reasoning is that if superoxide and hydrogen peroxide react with each other, they form one of the most active (i.e. dangerous) free radicals of all - hydroxyl radical, OH.

However, that is not the end of the story. Another expert, Dr. David G. Williams, has extensively researched this issue and considers the internal ingestion of H2O2 to be perfectly safe. He notes:

- *"A single atom of oxygen, however, is very reactive and is referred to as a free radical. Over the past several years, we've continually read that these free radicals are responsible for all types of ailments and even premature aging. What many writers seem to forget, however, is that our bodies create and use free radicals to destroy harmful bacteria, viruses, and fungi."*

In fact, the cells responsible for fighting infection and foreign invaders in the body (your white blood cells) make hydrogen peroxide and use it to oxidize any offending culprits. The intense bubbling you see when hydrogen peroxide comes in contact with a bacteria-laden cut or wound is the oxygen being released and bacteria being destroyed. The ability of our cells to produce hydrogen peroxide is essential for life. H2O2 is not some undesirable by-product or toxin, but instead a basic requirement for good health.
Ref: http://www.purehealthsystems.com/hydrogen-peroxide-2.html

Hydrogen peroxide is available in various strengths and grades:

3% Pharmaceutical Grade: This is the grade sold at your local drugstore or supermarket. This product is not recommended for internal use. It contains an assortment of stabilizers which shouldn't be ingested. Various stabilizers include: acetanilide, phenol, sodium stanate and tertrasodium phosphate.

6% Beautician Grade: This is used in beauty shops to color hair and is not recommended for internal use.

30% Reagent Grade: This is used for various scientific experimentation and also contains stabilizers. It is also not for internal use.

30% to 32% Electronic Grade: This is used to clean electronic parts and not for internal use.

35% Technical Grade: This is a more concentrated product than the Reagent Grade and differs slightly in that phosphorus is added to help neutralize any chlorine from the water used to dilute it.

8% and 35% Food Grade: This is used in the production of foods like cheese, eggs, and whey-containing products. It is also sprayed on the foil lining of aseptic packages containing fruit juices and milk products. THIS IS THE ONLY GRADE RECOMMENDED FOR INTERNAL USE...

90%: This is used as an oxygen source for rocket fuel.

Only [highly diluted] 8% or 35% Food Grade hydrogen peroxide is recommended for internal use [note: obviously his point is that only Food Grade hydrogen peroxide should be taken internally, there are lower concentrations than 35%]. At this concentration [i.e. 35%], however, hydrogen peroxide is a very strong oxidizer and **if not diluted,** it can be extremely dangerous or even fatal. Any concentrations over 10% can cause neurological reactions and damage to the upper gastrointestinal tract.
Ref: http://www.purehealthsystems.com/hydrogen-peroxide-2.html

Regardless of how hydrogen peroxide is used, it can be toxic if its concentration is too high. However, when diluted to theraputic levels it is totally safe for external use or I.V.s.

Ozone – Similar concern as with peroxide, ozone therapy must be done with a competent physician. Refer to http://www.oxygenhealingtherapies.com/intro_ozone.html for more information

Other dietary supplements helpful for Lyme patients include: bovine colostrums, lycopene and DHEA to improve growth hormone and other hormone deficiencies, the minerals magnesium and potassium, vitamin C, vitamin E (mixed tocopherols), and a good multi-vitamin that contains no retinyl palmitate form of vitamin A. Vitamin B12 helps deal with neuropathies. It can be taken sublingual (under the tongue) daily or preferably by subcutaneous weekly injections. Other supplements that will help to reduce inflammation and support the immune system include Borage and/or Evening Primrose oil, and DMAE. DMAE (dimethylaminoethanol) helps with fatigue caused by Lyme disease. Astragalus is an herb that is used for immune support.

Protecting the Nervous System from Neurotoxins

It is important to protect the peripheral and central nervous system from the toxins produced by borrelia. The following is a list of dietary supplements that are effective for this:

SAMe: S-adenosyl-L-methionine: The beneficial effects of SAMe supplementation are extensive because this nutrient is involved in so many metabolic processes, including its role in serving to detoxify cell membranes and synthesize neurotransmitters. From acting as an antioxidant to raising serotonin levels in the brain, SAMe is one of the most important compounds to come to the market. Studies on the use of SAMe in maintaining normal joint function are also promising.

Phosphadityl choline: Take 1 tablespoon of lecithin with each meal.

DMAE (dimethylaminoethanol) is a precursor to acetyl choline and has many benefits for CLD therapy.

B-vitamins: CLD patients need high doses of B-vitamins, especially B-6, **B-12**, and folic acid.

Anti-oxidant that are effective at protecting the nervous system include: pycnogenol, **grape seed extract**, bilberry, and **alpha lipoic acid**.

Detoxifying and Excreting the Toxins of Borrelia

Borrelia produce numerous toxic BLPs. These toxins are important because they trigger many harmful responses in the body including the inflammation that is damaging to healthy tissue, and cause the dysfunction of the immune system. These toxins are fat-soluble lipoproteins and are very difficult to rid the body of. The body normally detoxifies fat-soluble substances in the liver and excretes them from the bile. Unfortunately, the toxins appear to be reabsorbed from the gut and circulate back into the body.

Treatments designed to aid the body in eliminating these toxins is a very important part of a complete and comprehensive Lyme disease therapy.

Chlorella

- Very effective detoxifier
- Stimulates the immune system
- Contains growth factors that stimulate the regeneration of damaged tissues.

Bentonite: is a clay-like substance that attracts lipophilic compounds

Cholestyramine (Questran or Cholistad): a prescription that traps lipophilic compounds. Cholestyramine can cause constipation as a side effect.

Milk Thistle: Is probably the best herb that helps the liver detoxify and excrete bile.

Glutathione

Glutathione just may be our body's most powerful antioxidant; it plays an integral part in modulating (balancing) the immune response. It is manufactured by your body at adequate levels unless you are under higher than normal levels of stress, both emotional and chemical. The most common chemical stressors are dietary-induced, insulin surges from sugary, high-carb diets. Also common are hyper-immune, over-stimulations from food intolerances (largely precipitated by intestinal barrier compromises), chronic gastrointestinal infections from H-pylori, bad bacteria or parasites, hormonal imbalances and circadian rhythm disturbances, sleep deprivation, and autoimmune disorders.

Many people suffer from all of the above on a daily basis and also may smoke, drink too much, or even over train athletically, compounding an already precarious situation. Of course, CLD that has become an autoimmune disease itself is a significant stressor, further depleting the body's precious supply of glutathione.

In fact, I might go so far as to say it is difficult for the body to produce an autoimmune attack if the glutathione system is functioning properly.

Boosting glutathione levels though a liposomal topical cream, liposomal oral solution or intravenously—as glutathione taken orally by itself is fairly ineffective—is a key strategy in combating the damage of stress. However these levels can be quickly depleted if the body cannot recycle glutathione to keep the supply on hand to meet the many stressors.

Glutathione's job is to take the bullet

Before I can explain how glutathione recycling works, I first need to explain more about how specifically glutathione protects us. Glutathione is like the bodyguard or Secret Service agent whose loyalty is so deep that she will jump in front of a bullet to save the life of the one she protects. When there is enough of the proper form of glutathione in the body to "take the bullet", no inflammatory response occurs. However when glutathione becomes depleted it triggers a destructive inflammatory process.

Glutathione recycling explained

Glutathione *recycling* is a separate function from just boosting glutathione levels through a liposomal cream, liposomal oral solution, intravenously, a nebulizer, a suppository, or other means. These forms of glutathione delivery will help one's antioxidant status but they do not raise levels of glutathione *inside the cells*. Glutathione is the main antioxidant for mitochondria, the little factories inside each cell that convert nutrients into energy. Some cells have more mitochondria than others depending on the cell's function. This is important because an autoimmune disease destroys the mitochondria in the affected cells, thus causing tissue destruction, and glutathione protects these mitochondria.

Reduced glutathione versus oxidized glutathione

But not just any form of glutathione does this—it needs to be *reduced glutathione*. There are two main forms of glutathione in the body: reduced glutathione (GSH) and oxidized glutathione (GSSG).

Reduced glutathione, or GSH, is the bodyguard who "takes the hit" from free radicals that damage cells. Free radicals are molecules that are unstable because they have unpaired electrons and are looking for another electron to steal in order to become stable. They steal electrons from the mitochondria, thus destroying them and causing inflammation and degeneration.

However when there's plenty of GSH in the cell, the GSH sacrifice themselves to the free radicals—throwing themselves in front of the bullet—in order to protect the mitochondria. Thus the GSH ends up with an unpaired electron and becomes unstable, at which point it becomes GSSG, or oxidized glutathione, which is technically a free radical itself.

Doesn't this make GSSG dangerous to the cell then? When there is sufficient glutathione in the cell, the unstable GSSG naturally pairs with available glutathione in the cell with the help of an enzyme called glutathione reductase, returning back to its reduced glutathione state so it's ready for action once again.

The key thing to remember is that two enzymes play important roles in these processes:

- *Glutathione peroxidase* triggers the reaction of GSH to GSSG, which is when glutathione "takes the hit" to spare the cell

- *Glutathione reductase* triggers the conversion of GSSG back to useable GSH.

These enzymes come into consideration when we look at how to support the glutathione system nutritionally.

The link between poor glutathione recycling and CLD autoimmune disease

Studies show a direct correlation between a breakdown in the glutathione system and all of the autoimmune diseases. The ability to constantly take oxidized glutathione and recycle it back to reduced glutathione is critical for managing autoimmunity.

Fortunately studies also show various botanicals, nutritional compounds, and their cofactors have been shown to activate glutathione reductase and the synthesis of reduced glutathione. By boosting this enzyme and supplementing glutathione levels we can increase glutathione levels and glutathione recycling to quench inflammation once it starts, or, even better, to prevent inflammation in the first place.

Studies have also shown that efficient glutathione recycling helps boost the TH-3 system (also called the T-regulatory system), the branch of the immune system that helps balance the TH-1 and TH-2 systems and prevent autoimmune reactivity. (I explain TH-1 and TH-2 systems of immunity in my book, "Help My Body is Killing Me" available as a free download at www.upperroomwellness.com or at www.amazon.com). Proper glutathione activity not only helps protect cells, research shows it also modulates cell proliferation and immunity, and helps tissues recover from damage.

Glutathione recycling helps repair leaky gut

Good glutathione recycling helps tame autoimmune diseases in another way. One thing I have found universal in all my autoimmune patients is poor gut integrity. They all suffer from some degree of leaky gut and repairing the gut is vital to the recovery process. Studies show glutathione may play an important role in gut barrier function and the prevention of intestinal inflammation.

A compromised glutathione recycling system can worsen intestinal destruction—the person with multiple food sensitivities and a gut that never heals may be victim of this mechanism. Although repairing a leaky gut is vital to taming an autoimmune response, we can see now glutathione recycling is another vital piece to the puzzle of restoring gut health.

Supporting glutathione recycling

So how do we support glutathione recycling? The first thing is to reduce the stressors depleting this vital system. The bulk of my thyroid book is devoted to this: balancing blood sugar, addressing food intolerances, restoring gut health, and managing adrenal function are foundational.

Other considerations are neurotransmitter imbalances and hormonal imbalances, which may require specialized guidance from a qualified health care practitioner. And of course making any lifestyle changes you can, such as getting enough sleep, paring down an overactive schedule, making exercise a priority each day, creating time to do things you love, and so on.

Once you have addressed these factors (which for many people can actually take care of the problem) and autoimmune dysfunction persists, then boosting glutathione recycling may be necessary. Below I cover the basic botanicals and nutritional compounds researchers have found support glutathione recycling pathways. (I like a product from Apex Energetics called **Glutathione Recycler**)

- N-acetyl-cysteine (NAC): NAC is a key compound to glutathione activity. It is rapidly metabolized into intracellular glutathione.

- Alpha-lipoic acid (ALA): ALA directly recycles and extends the metabolic life spans of vitamin C, glutathione, and coenzyme Q10, and it indirectly renews vitamin E, all of which are necessary for glutathione recycling.

- L-glutamine: Research has shown that l-glutamine is important for the generation of glutathione. It is transported into the cell, converted to glutamate, and readily available to intracellular glutathione synthesis.

- Selenium: Selenium is a trace element nutrient that serves as the essential cofactor for the enzyme glutathione peroxidase, which converts GSH to GSSG so glutathione can "take the hit" by free radicals to spare cells.

- Cordyceps: Cordyceps has been shown to activate both glutathione and peroxidase synthesis in the body. It has also been shown to protect cells by engaging the glutathione enzyme cycle.

- Gotu kola (Centella Asiatica): Research has clearly demonstrated that oral intake of gotu kola rapidly and dramatically increases the activity and amount of glutathione peroxidase and the quantity of glutathione.

- Milk thistle (Silybum marianum): Milk thistle has been shown to significantly increase glutathione, increase superoxide dismutase (another powerful antioxidant) activity, and positively influence the ratios of reduced and oxidized glutathione.

Taken together these botanicals and compounds activate the glutathione peroxidase and reductase enzymes that promote a healthy glutathione recycling system.

For people with severe leaky gut issues I suggest they take these compounds as they work on repairing leaky gut. Also, it's important to use these in conjunction with a liposomal glutathione cream discussed in the book. These compounds work more on recycling glutathione than boosting overall levels. This way the glutathione you do take, whether through a cream, an IV, a nasal spray, or other method is assured to stay in your body longer and get inside your cells where they can do their best work.

Glutathione recycling is imperative to taming autoimmune disease

Promoting glutathione recycling helps protect cell mitochondria, enhance tissue recovery, modulate an imbalance between TH-1 and TH-2, and boost immune regulation. The overall effect is to dampen both the autoimmune reaction and damage to body tissue. It also helps body tissue and the intestinal tract regenerate and recover. Keeping overall glutathione levels up by supporting glutathione recycling helps buffer the body's cells from the many stressors hurled at us each day.

Other practitioners and I have witnessed patients rebuild their glutathione recycling system. As a result they are much less or no longer sensitive to chemicals around them, they have fewer autoimmune flare-ups, and they recover much faster from their flare-ups.

NOTE: See my formula to make your own Liposomal Glutathione oral solution in the appendix at the back of this book.

Hemp Oil

Medicinal Cannabis Extract

Though currently illegal in the United States, Cannabis Extract Medicine, also known as "hemp oil" when referring to the type pioneered by Rick Simpson, is a concentrated formulation of cannabis that is ingested orally. Do NOT confuse this with hemp seed oil – that is completely different and does NOT work, as hemp seed contains NO active THC. By ingesting hemp oil over a three to six month period, many diseases, including cancer and chronic Lyme disease can either be cured or completely controlled. This is possible because cannabis medicine works fundamentally through the endocannabinoid system, the super-regulatory system of the body that maintains homeostasis in the other systems.

There are literally hundreds upon hundreds of scientific studies showing that cannabinoids like tetrahydrocannabinol (THC) and cannabidiol (CBD), as well as whole plant formulations, are effective against nearly any disease you can think of. According to Dr. Robert Ramer and Dr. Burkhard Hinz of the University of Rostock in Germany medical marijuana can be an effective treatment for cancer. Their research was published in the Journal of the National Cancer Institute Advance Access on December 25th of 2007 in a paper entitled Inhibition of Cancer Cell Invasion by Cannabinoids via Increased Expression of Tissue Inhibitor of Matrix Metalloproteinases-1. (1)

The biggest contribution of this breakthrough discovery, is that the expression of TIMP-1 was shown to be stimulated by cannabinoid receptor activation and to mediate the anti-invasive effect of cannabinoids. Prior to now the cellular mechanisms underlying this effect were unclear and the relevance of the findings to the behavior of tumor cells in vivo remains to be determined.

The science for the use of hemp oil is credible, specific fact-based, and is documented in detail. (1) There is absolutely no reason to not legalize medical marijuana and create an immediate production and distribution of THC hemp oil to cancer patients. Unfortunately we live in a world populated with governments and medical henchmen who would rather see people die cruel deaths then have access to a safe and effect cancer drug.

Meanwhile the Food and Drug Administration approved Genentech's best-selling drug, Avastin, as a treatment for breast cancer, in a decision, according to the New York Times, "that appeared to lower the threshold somewhat for approval of certain cancer drugs. The big question was whether it was enough for a drug temporarily to stop cancer from worsening — as Avastin had done in a clinical trial — or was it necessary for a drug to enable patients to live longer, which Avastin had failed to do. Oncologists and patient advocates were divided, in part because of the drug's sometimes severe side effects."

The differences between Avastin and hemp oil are huge. First Avastin will earn Genentech hundreds of millions where THC hemp oil will earn no one anything. Second there are no severe or even mild side effects to taking hemp oil and lastly it is not a temporary answer but a real solution. Certainly hemp oil will ensure a longer life. So is life in a greed-driven nation that approves medication based on profits and dismisses natural cures based on their ability to lessen pharmaceutical income.

Here is Rick Simpson's testimony on Hemp Oil and Cancer:

Rick Simpson's BACKGROUND (2)

Would you please describe how you came to discover the cure for cancer?

I am just one of many who have found a way to cure cancer. A radio broadcast told me that T.H.C. (tetrahydracannabinol) kills cancer so I do not claim that it was me who found the cure. I may be the first to have people ingesting hemp oil and applying it topically to treat their cancers and other conditions but I do not feel that it was really me who found the cure. What I did do was find the proper way to use this wonderful medicine. As often as I could, I provided the medicine free of charge and then I openly reported my findings to the government and the public, expecting that the right thing would be done.

How did you find out about THC being effective to treat cancer?

In 1972 I watched my 25 year-old cousin die a horrible death from cancer. About three years later I heard a report on our local radio station CKDH in Amherst, Nova Scotia. The announcer was laughing like a fool when he gave the report so I did not know whether or not to take the report seriously. He stated that T.H.C. (the active substance in marijuana) has been found to kill cancer cells. After this report I heard nothing more on this subject so I assumed that it must have been some kind of joke. About 30 years later I found out that the report was true and it was from the Medical School of Virginia study done in 1974.

In 1997 I suffered a head injury that left me with Post Concussion Syndrome. The chemicals the medical system gave me did nothing for my condition but make me worse with the side effects. Then, in 1998, I saw an episode of The Nature of Things entitled "Reefer Madness II". Dr. David Suzuki interviewed people who were smoking hemp for their medical conditions and the results were amazing. After watching the show I purchased some hemp to see if it would help my condition. Post-Concussion Syndrome can affect people in different ways; some wind up with severe migraines… in my case I wound up with what can only be termed as migraine noise. It's like having a tuning fork gone mad in your head that you cannot silence. If this condition persists the noise takes over your life and you get very little rest. When I smoked hemp for my condition it relaxed me and allowed me to get more sleep. Smoking hemp did not take the noise in my head away but it did make the condition much easier to live with.

I asked many doctors for a prescription for hemp but was refused. They would use excuses like "it's still under study" and "hemp is bad for the lungs" or some other such nonsense.

About 1999 I asked my family doctor what he thought about me making the essential oil from the hemp plant and ingesting it as a medication as opposed to smoking it. My doctor said that ingesting the oil would be much more medicinal but still would not provide me with a prescription. By 2002 the medical system had written me off. I was told by my doctor that they had tried every medication at their disposal but none of them helped me so I was on my own. The doctor knew very well that the only medication that helped me was hemp. He also knew that I would be classified as a criminal if I was caught using hemp for my condition, but still he would provide no prescription, the same as all the other doctors I had asked. Can you imagine, I had worked for 32 years and had never had a drug charge in my life? Now due to my need for this medication for my condition, suddenly I am now a criminal because they would not give me the legal right to use this medicine. Needless to say, all of this left a very bad taste in my mouth.

You said it had cured your skin cancer in no time – how many days did it take? Did it come back? Does it usually come back?

In late 2002 my doctor examined three areas on my body which he suspected were skin cancer. One was close to my right eye, another was on my left cheek, and there was another area on my chest. In January

2003 I went in to have the cancer close to my right eye removed. I was to go in at a later date and have the other two areas taken care of. About a week after the surgery I was examining the area where they had removed the cancer, when suddenly the report I had heard on the radio 30 years before popped back into my mind. The report had stated that THC kills cancer cells. I knew the oil that I produced was full of THC so I thought why not put some oil on the other two cancers and see what happens. I applied the oil and covered it with a bandage and left it in place for four days. During this time I felt nothing so I assumed that the oil was not working. Imagine my surprise after removing the bandages and seeing nothing but pink skin – the cancer was gone! Within seven weeks the cancers close to my right eye that they had removed surgically returned. I applied the oil and a bandage to this area and in four days it too was completely healed. I performed these treatments on myself in the winter of 2003. I have never applied oil to these areas again and the cancer has never returned.

PROTOCOL

Is there a protocol for the treatment?

There is a protocol, and it should be followed to ensure that the treatment is effective. Small amounts of oil can be used to treat skin cancer or the oil can be vaporized and inhaled directly in the lungs to treat lung conditions in addition to ingesting. Also, the oil may be absorbed into the body if used in the form of a suppository.

To treat internal cancers the oil must be ingested. I usually start people out with three or four doses a day, about the size of half a grain of dry rice. The only time I would suggest that people start with a heavier dose would be if there was a lot of pain involved with their condition. Often times many of these folks are already addicted to dangerous and deadly pain medications. The object in such cases is to get these people off these dangerous drugs and to replace them with hemp oil to ease their pain.

I suggest that about every four days the dosage be increased slowly until the patient has worked their way up to taking a gram a day. At this point most people continue taking a gram a day until they are cured. In more than one case I have seen people take the full 60 gram treatment and cure their cancer in a month.

How is hemp oil usually tolerated?

We all have different tolerances for different medications so I encourage people to stay in their own comfort zone when dosing themselves with the oil. Most people's tolerances build very quickly and on average a normal person usually takes about 90 days to ingest the 60 gram treatment. 60 grams seems to be able to cure most cancers but people who have suffered extensive damage from chemo and radiation may require more to undo the damage the medical system has left behind. For some external skin conditions, etc., where full strength oil is not required, the oil can be mixed with skin creams and salves. Mixing hemp oil with facial creams does wonders for the complexion if you give yourself a facial with it, also it should be used in such things as suntan lotions.

We know from our experience with hemp salves and our cosmetics that hemp is basically a cure-all. Can you confirm this?

History calls hemp a panacea, which means cure all. From my experience, seeing hemp oil used for various medical conditions, I too call hemp a cure all. Hemp is useful in the treatment of practically any disease or condition; it promotes full-body healing. From our experience the oil is also very beneficial for most skin conditions; it can be mixed with skin creams or even suntan lotion. Wouldn't it be nice to go out in the sun and not have to worry about skin cancer?

CANCER

What is hemp oil good for?

From my experience, the oil is effective in the treatment of all types of skin cancers, and the same holds true for internal cancers and other medical conditions.

Which types of cancer is this best for? Are you aware of any types that this will not help with?

Hemp oil seems to work on all types of cancer and I am not aware of any type of cancer that it would not be effective for. I have heard about a study that claims that THC can cause a certain type of cancer; I can only say that this study must be flawed. Put simply, cancer is just mutating cells; THC kills mutating cells. So how can THC produce the very cells that it is so good at killing? If you are looking for treatments that can cause cancer, look no further than chemo and radiation; both of these so-called "treatments" are very carcinogenic. In other words they can and do cause cancer. Even a CT scan exposes the body to a massive dose of radiation. Radiation causes cells to mutate, and that is what cancer is... mutating cells.

When people come to me with cancer of course I recommend the oil, but along with hemp oil I also suggest that they change their diets. Protein from fruits and vegetables fight cancer. Animal protein promotes cancer. So it is best to stay away from animal protein. I also suggest mega-doses of vitamins, especially vitamin C; this is known as Gerson therapy, and I am a total believer in it. Also there are many other natural things a person can do to fight cancer. Bringing the body's Ph up with lemon juice and baking soda and water is very beneficial (two to three times a day, there is no set dosage, just mix it as strong as the patient can drink it). Also I have heard good reports about wheat grass being effective for cancer. I am also convinced that B17 can be very beneficial for cancer sufferers. Every day I eat the seeds from two apples. Like apricots, apple seeds contain B17, also known as laetrile. B17 in its own right has a good track record with cancer. Many people whom I provided the oil to did not change their diets or anything else but were still cured with the oil. From my point of view, anyone with cancer should be doing everything they possibly can to optimize their chance of survival. So by all means, take hemp oil for your cancer, but do not ignore other natural beneficial treatments.

What is the success rate for cancer patients?

Cancer can be reversed in roughly 75% of people who have been badly damaged by the medical system; if they are willing to take the treatment properly. However, there is about 1 in 4 who has been so badly damaged that no matter what you do you cannot save them. Even if you can cure the cancer, in the end the damage from the chemo and radiation will kill them. These people are not dying from cancer; they are dying from the so-called "medical treatments" they receive from the medical system.

How many people that you know of have cured themselves with the oil? Have you ever failed to cure someone (because it did not work for him/her)?

I have provided the oil to well over 2,500 people over the last seven years. Due to the illegal status of hemp oil I do not keep records but it is safe to say I have seen hundreds of people cured with external and internal cancers, plus a great number of other conditions.

When people come to me with a diagnoses of cancer and they have refused to take chemotherapy or radiation it is almost a given that they can be cured, unless they wait until they are at death's door to take the treatment. We had one gentleman about four years ago who was in the hospital and was given 24 hours to live. The doctors refused to give him the oil, so his son did it. The very next day this man discharged himself from the hospital, went home and stayed on the oil. About fourteen months later this 83 year-old veteran did die, but not from lung cancer; he died from a pre-existing heart condition that he had for years. During the fourteen extra months that he had lived, he enjoyed a good quality of life and he died in his sleep with no pain. Isn't that better than dying in a hospital, drowning in your own fluid from lung cancer? I tell everyone that comes to me one thing… the oil will either save your life or it will ease your way out. If you do die, you will die with dignity and not full of such drugs as morphine.

Are some people more difficult to cure than others?

People who are the hardest to cure are the ones who have allowed themselves to be severely damaged by the medical system. Chemotherapy and radiation are both carcinogenic treatments, in other words they cause cancer. Chemotherapy and radiation can reduce the size of a tumor, but in the end usually all such treatments do is spread the cancer.

When hemp oil is ingested as a cancer medication, the THC in the oil causes a buildup of a fat molecule called ceramide. When ceramide comes in contact with cancer cells it causes programmed cell death of the cancer cells while doing no harm to healthy cells. This is the way it was explained in the scientific research we have studied. But with the help of a good friend named Batya Stark, I have developed a new theory.

A few months ago, Batya sent me some reports about the pineal gland and melatonin. The significance of the information she put in front of me was undeniable. So between Batya and I, we started connecting the dots. And this is what we concluded. Fluoride and a great deal of the chemicals doctors provide plus other we come into contact with often harm the ability of the pineal gland to produce melatonin. Melatonin is the greatest antioxidant known to man and it travels to every cell in the body. The pineal gland and the melatonin it produces plays a very dramatic role in maintaining good health and indeed has a lot to do with the aging process.

With the function of the pineal gland impaired, its ability to produce melatonin is greatly diminished. It has been found that cancer sufferers have reduced melatonin levels. It has also been scientifically proven that just smoking hemp can raise melatonin levels a great deal. Now just think of what eating the raw unburned oil would do melatonin levels. From what I understand, the oil causes the pineal gland to go into overdrive and subsequently melatonin levels go through the roof. And this at least in part is what we think causes the wonderful effect this medication has on so many conditions. If the pineal gland is producing vast amounts of melatonin, it does no harm to the body. In such a situation, the illness of disease that has been plaguing the patient are brought under control and often completely healed. When you work with properly produced hemp medicines, you soon realize the word "incurable" means very little.

1. *SPAIN STUDY CONFIRMS CANNABIS OIL CURES CANCER WITHOUT SIDE EFFECTS, October 10, 2012 · by thscollapsereport in Healthcare*

2. *http://phoenixtears.ca/tag/legal, Rick Simpson*

Hyperthermia

Borrelia prefer temperatures below that of the body. Using hot showers, baths, or infra-red saunas at temperatures of up to 104 degrees F for 20-30 minutes daily to raise the body temperature is a helpful therapy for treating CLD. Borrelia species are especially sensitive to the combination of other therapies and heat. Raising the body temperature also dilates the peripheral circulation and increases the permeability of the blood vessels throughout the body. These physiological changes assist in the delivery of antibiotics to all areas of the body increasing the amount of antibiotics able to penetrate and reach the borrelia.

Ref: Southern Medical Journal: October 1995 - Volume 88 - Issue 10 - ppg S142 Conjoint Meeting with the American Society of Clinical Hyperthermic Oncology

The History of Energy Medicine

Everything is ENERGY

"The cell is a machine driven by energy. It can thus be approached by studying matter, or by studying energy. In every culture and in every medical tradition before ours, healing was accomplished by moving energy."

----Albert Szent-Gyorgyi, Nobel Laureate in Medicine

All cells are capable of receiving a countless number of frequencies that are stored within the cytoplasm of each cell, which itself, consists of H2O. Hydrogen and Oxygen hold the electromagnetic charges, and the cellular memory is then processed within the DNA of each cell. Vital life energy (Bio-energy) fills every cell within the human body, which controls all metabolic processes, including biochemical changes that occur within the cells. It controls the utilization of nutritional substances, and the functioning of all body systems including the immune system.

We predicate that during periods of stress, be it physical or mental stress, this increases the cell's state of vulnerability to discordant frequencies (stressors). For example, electromagnetic fields such as mobile phones, microwaves, computers, household wiring etc., can enter cells through the Integral membrane proteins in the cell membrane and store in the cytoplasm, altering the cell's homeostasis. Cells are most vulnerable during periods of stress: the greater the stress, the greater the incidence of acquiring homeostatic imbalance. By recognizing discordant frequencies within cells, the body is more capable of achieving homeostasis. Every disease state and pathogen has its associated harmonic and disharmonic frequencies. Generally speaking, harmonic frequencies maintain health (homeostasis); promote growth and healing, while disharmonic frequencies produce illness and death (homeostatic imbalance).

New research introduces a radical understanding of cell science. New biology concepts reveal that human beings control their genome rather than being controlled by it. It is now recognized that environmental frequencies and more specifically, our perception or interpretation of the environment, directly controls the activity of our genes. This new paradigm of "bio-electrical interaction" has given us a better understanding of how the human body uses energy to heal itself and regulate its activities. It has also enabled science to reevaluate previously discarded medical therapies and to explore new ones based on this interaction.

During the 1990s, three Nobel Prize winners in medicine in the field of advanced medical research revealed that the primary function of DNA lies not in protein synthesis, as widely believed, but in electromagnetic energy reception and transmission. Less than three percent of DNA's function is in protein formulation; more than ninety percent of the DNA functions in the realm of bioelectric signaling. One might say that electromagnetism is fundamentally responsible for all life, and everything in the physical universe. It is also in the spiritual force or energy that gives rise to all matter.

From: Bioelectromagnetic Healing, its History and a Rationale for its Use

Thomas F. Valone, Integrity Research Institute, 1220 L Street NW, Suite 100-232 Washington DC 20005, www.IntegrityResearchInstitute.org

"Bioelectromagnetics (BEMs) is the study of the effect of electromagnetic fields on biological systems.1 Though electromagnetic fields have sometimes been associated with potential for harm to the body, there are many BEM instruments and devices re-emerging in the 21st century, based on high voltage Tesla coils, that apparently bring beneficial health improvements to human organisms. The Tesla coil class of therapy devices constitute pulsed electromagnetic fields (PEMF) that deliver broadband, wide spectrum, nonthermal photons and electrons deep into biological tissue. *Here listed are the two most prominent players and possibly the most important medical scientists of our day:*

Nikola Tesla

In 1895, the Niagara Falls Power Company opened for the first time and within a year, sent alternating current (AC) to Buffalo, NY, twenty-five miles away, thanks to Nikola Tesla AC generators. Cities throughout the world followed suit and made commercial AC power available to the general public, even miles from the power generating station. As a result, Tesla's high voltage coil devices, which were powered by AC, started to become widely known and applied.

In 1898, Tesla published a paper that he read at the eighth annual meeting of the American Electro-Therapeutic Association in Buffalo, NY entitled, "High Frequency Oscillators for Electro-Therapeutic and Other Purposes."2 He states that "One of the early observed and remarkable features of the high frequency currents, and one which was chiefly of interest to the physician, was their apparent harmlessness which made it possible to pass relatively great amounts of electrical energy through the body of a person without causing pain or serious discomfort." Coils up to three feet in diameter were used for magnetically treating the body without contact, though ten to a hundred thousand volts were present "between the first and last turn." Preferably, Tesla describes using spheres of brass covered with two inches of insulating wax for contacting the patient, while unpleasant shocks were prevented. Tesla concludes correctly that bodily "tissues are condensers" in the 1898 paper, which is the basic component (dielectric) for an equivalent circuit only recently developed for the human body.3 In fact, the relative permittivity for tissue at any frequency from ELF (10 Hz-100 Hz) through RF (10 kHz– 100 MHz) exceeds most commercially available dielectrics on the market.4 This unique property of the human body indicates an inherent adaptation and perhaps innate compatibility toward the presence of high voltage electric fields, probably due to the high transmembrane potential already present in cellular tissue.

Tesla also indicates that the after-effect from his coil treatment "was certainly beneficial" but that an hour exposure was too strong to be used frequently. This has been found to be still true today with the Tesla coil therapy devices. On September 6, 1932, at a seminar presented by the American Congress of Physical Therapy, held in New York, Dr. Gustave Kolischer announced: "Tesla's high-frequency electrical currents are bringing about highly beneficial results in dealing with cancer, surpassing anything that could be accomplished with ordinary surgery."

Other scientists followed. Georges Lakhovsky, during the early to middle part of the last century produced various broad band multiple wave oscillator circuits that similarly to Tesla's circuits, produced broad-band (wide spectrum of frequencies) ultrasound in human tissue. Dr. Albert Abrams, also in the first part of last century, developed various electrical oscillation circuits that supplied electrodes connected to the human body with complex voltage oscillation patterns that produced broad band ultrasound in human tissue. One of the most notable persons was John Crane, an associate and business partner of Dr. Rife during the last twenty years of Rife's life. John Crane popularized the use of electrodes applying a voltage square wave to the human body. Crane's voltage square wave generator, when tuned to specific frequencies, was able to achieve many of the curative results as the "Rife Frequency Instrument". Since John Crane, others have come forward with essentially "spin-offs" on the voltage square wave applied to the skin by electrodes method. Some devices use high voltage surges applied to the body through inert gas discharge tubes.

Royal Raymond Rife

In 1934, the University of Southern California appointed a Special Medical Research Committee to study 16 terminal cancer patients from Pasadena County Hospital that would be treated with mitogenic impulse-wave technology, developed by Royal Raymond Rife. After four months the Medical Research Committee reported that all 16 of the formerly-terminal patients appeared cured.

Rife's high voltage gas tube device was designed, with the aid of his unique microscope, by experimentally witnessing the effects on microbes and bacteria, finding what he believed were the particular frequencies that resonated with their destruction. "In 1938, Rife made his most public announcement. In a two-part article written by Newall Jones of the San Diego Evening Tribune (May 6 & 11), Rife said, 'We do not wish at this time to claim that we have "cured" cancer, or any other disease, for that matter. But we can say that these waves, or this ray, as the frequencies might be called, have been shown to possess the power of devitalizing disease organisms, of "killing" them, when tuned to an exact wave length, or frequency, for each organism. This applies to the organisms both in their free state and, with certain exceptions, when they are in living tissues.'"10

"He had the backing in his day - this was in the 1930's - of such eminent people as Kendall, a professor of pathology at Northwestern University and Millbank Johnson, M.D., who was on his board, along with many other medical men, when he began to treat people with this new 'ray emitter.'... There were articles written on the Rife technique... in the Journal for the Medical Society of California and other medical journals. Suddenly, Rife came under the glassy eye of Morris Fishbein of the AMA and things began to happen very quickly. Rife was put on trial for having invented a 'phony' medical cure. The trial lasted a long time."11

In 1953, Rife published his cancer report in book form, History of the Development of a Successful Treatment for Cancer and Other Virus, Bacteria and Fungi.12 A turning point occurred in 1958, when the State of California Public Health Department conducted a hearing which ordered the testing of Rife's Frequency Instrument. The Palo Alto Detection Lab, the Kalbfeld Lab, the UCLA Medical Lab, and the San Diego Testing Lab all participated in the evaluation procedure. "All reported that it was safe to use. Nevertheless, the AMA Board, under Dr. Malcolm Merrill, the Director of Public Health, declared it unsafe and banned it from the market."13

In 1961, after a trial with an AMA doctor as the foreman of the jury, John F. Crane, the new owner of the Rife Virus Microscope Institute, spent three years in jail, ostensibly for using the Frequency Instrument on people, though no specific criminal intent had been proven. In 1965, he attempted to obtain approval from the California Board of Public Health for use of the Frequency Instrument. "On November 17, 1965, the Department of Public Health replied that Crane had not shown that the device was safe or 'effective in use.'"14

From 1968 to 1983, Dr. Livingston-Wheeler treated approximately 10,000 patients with the Rife Frequency Instrument, at her University of Southern California clinic, with an 80% success rate. In 1972, Dr. Livingston-Wheeler published Cancer:

A New Breakthrough in which she "condemned the National Cancer Institute for its misuse of money [$500 million in 13 years], the corrupt handling of public health responsibilities, and its use of people [100,000 cancer patients] as guinea pigs for a 'surgery-radiation- chemotherapy' program dictated by special interests." Her last book on The Conquest of Cancer was published in 1984 in which she celebrates the European acceptance of the Rife discoveries but complains about the situation in the U.S.

All of these distinguished scientists, back in 1958, had been carrying on significant research in the biological and immunological treatment of cancer for years. It is still only now that the United States orthodoxy is beginning to catch up. Because of the suppressive actions of the American Cancer Society, the American Medical Association, and the Food and Drug Administration, our people have not had the advantage of the European research.

This work has been ignored because certain powerful individuals backed by large monetary grants can become the dictators of research and suppress all work that does not promote their interests or that may present a threat to their prestige.

Rife died in 1971, mostly of a broken heart."

1 Bioelectromagnetics Society (founded 1978), 120 W. Church St., Frederick MD 21701. 301-663-4252

www.bioelectromagnetics.org

2 Tesla, N (1898) "High Frequency Oscillators for Electro-Therapeutic and Other Purposes," The Electrical Engineer, Vol. XXVI, No. 550, Nov. 17, p.477

3 Polk, C., and E. Postow, (1986) Handbook of Biological Effects of Electromagnetic Fields, CRC Press, p. 58

4 Fink, D.D., (1975) "Dielectric Constant and Loss Factor for Several Dielectrics," Electrical Engineer's Handbook, p. 6-36

5 Manning, Clark A. and L. J. Vanrenen, Bioenergetic Medicines East and West, North Atlantic Books, Berkeley, 1988, p. 43

6 Douglass, W. C. Into the Light—The Exciting Story of the Life-Saving Breakthrough Therapy of the Age, Second Opinion Pub., Atlanta, 1996, p. 269

7 Lakhovsky, Georges. "Curing Cancer with Ultra Radio Frequencies," Radio News, February, 1925, p. 1282-1283.

8 Grotz, Toby, and B. Hillstead. "Frequency Analysis of the Lakhovsky Multiple Wave Oscillator from 20 Hz to 20 GHz," Proceedings of the US Psychotronics Association Convention, Portland, OR, July, 1983

9 Bird, Christopher. "The Politics Of Science: A Background On Energy Medicine," Energetic Processes: Interaction Between Matter, Energy & Consciousness, Volume I, Xlibris Press, Philadelphia, 2001, p. 226 10 Lynes, Barry. The Cancer Cure That Worked: Fifty Years of Suppression, Marcus Books, Queensville, Ontario, 1987, p. 103

11 Bird, p. 227

12 Rife, Royal Raymond. History of the Development of a Successful Treatment for Cancer and Other Virus, Bacteria and Fungi. Rife Virus Microscope Institute, San Diego, CA, 1953

13 Lynes, p.129

14 Ibid., p. 133

15 Williams, R. M. "The Handbook of Rife Frequency Healing: Holistic Technology for Cancer and Other Diseases by Nina Silver, PhD." TOWNSEND LETTER FOR DOCTORS AND PATIENTS (2003): 121-122.

The Rife Machine

Rife machines are electronic devices that produce varying frequencies of energy (similar to a microwave, but at frequencies not harmful to the body). This energy penetrate the tissues of the body and cause the spiral-shaped Borrelia to resonate so much that the integrity of the bacteria is disrupted; weakening and even killing them. This is an effective means for killing borrelia and is supported by the production of herx reactions in Lyme patients after Rife treatments, while non-infected individuals don't experience the herx reactions when exposed to Rife treatment.

Rife machines are named after Royal Raymond Rife, born in 1888 in Elkhorn, Nebraska. From the 1920's through to his death in 1971 he lived and worked in San Diego, California. Rife real claim to fame came from two specific inventions (although he had many others). One was a super microscope allegedly capable of resolving objects below the Abbe limit, and with magnification claimed to be as high as 31,000 times. The second invention was an electromagnetic therapy device consisting of a light transmitter feeding a plasma tube (Tesla tube) which was claimed to kill specific pathogenic microorganisms at specific frequencies. It was claimed that in 1932 Rife succeeded in isolating a "filter-passing" microorganism (later referred to as the BX virus) that was a cause of cancer. And in 1934 it was further claimed that Rife succeeded in curing several cases of cancer in real patients by targeting this microorganism with his light frequency machine. The Rife technology was dismissed by the American Medical Association as quackery and was suppressed by various organizations and American federal agencies. This took place at the same time that the FDA and AMA went on their witch-hunt, driving many successful clinicians who were not using standard pharmaceutical agents to close their doors or move out of the country. Rife just quit and retreated, a broken man.

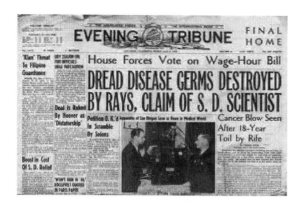

"Royal Raymond Rife was a man whose microscope, frequency instrument, and support of pleomorphism are still controversial today. With hopes of seeing where Mr. Rife's house once stood, I drove over to the location but could find nothing but a sign that read, "Chatsworth Blvd." I drove back and forth on Chatsworth Boulevard. There was no longer a 2500 Chatsworth Boulevard. There was nothing to indicate that, possibly, at this address, a "cure for cancer" was found by a man who began researching cancer in 1920 and, by 1932, had isolated the cancer "virus." In 1934, he opened a clinic that successfully cured 16 of 16 cases within 3 months. He developed an optical microscope that had a magnifying resolution that still surpasses any built today except for the electron microscope. He did not use fixed specimens. All of his observations were based on living specimens. He was able to isolate what he considered to be the cancer virus, which he injected into hundreds of laboratory mice that subsequently developed cancer. He found that the "cancer virus" could be destroyed by the use of electromagnetic radiation and proceeded to design an apparatus that did so (Lynes, 2001)."   - *Great Revolutionary Leaders of Alternative Medicine: A Fascinating Journey Back in Time*
RICHARD C. NIEMTZOW, M.D., Ph.D., M.P.H.

"Mr. Rife's discoveries, in my opinion, were buried by others' professional jealousy, greed, and ignorance. He was too far ahead of his time. Because many scientists did not understand what he developed,

they did their best to ignore it." - Barry Lyons, author of The Cancer Cure
That Worked

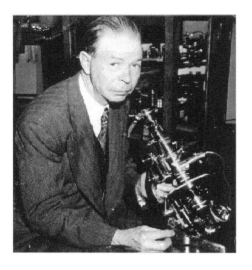

Rife believed that ***different species of life have their own
electromagnetic "signature"*** - a pattern of oscillation based on its
individual genetic chemical blueprint. His theories have been confirmed
by quantum physics though modern medicine ignores the healing
abilities connected to tapping those frequencies. Rife discovered that
viruses, bacteria, and parasites are particularly sensitive to their own
specific "bio frequencies" and could be destroyed by intensifying those
frequencies until they literally explode... like an intense musical note
that can shatter a wine glass! While cell walls of single-celled organisms
tend to be less stable and lyse when bombarded with their own or
similar frequencies, hitting human body cells with their own frequencies
does nothing but help. In order to "explode" the microbes, Rife invented
a "frequency beam ray" machine, similar to what we now call a Rife
Machine.

As Christopher Bird reported regarding bacterium/viruses, "...many
lethal (disease) those of tuberculosis, typhoid, leprosy . . . appeared to
disintegrate or 'blow- up' in the field of his microscope."

Use this link to view a number of informative videos on Rife:

http://www.rife.de/rife-related-videos.html

Types of Rife Machines

We have personally used all of the top selling Rife machines on the market. Currently I use two different types in my office, the Light Beam Generator and the Truerife (www.truerife.com). I would ONLY recommend the Truerife for anyone with Lyme disease! As a matter of fact, I will NO LONGER accept a CLD patient without them committing to purchase a Truerife machine. We include a fully programmed machine with every CLD and cancer patient that starts care with us – obviously I am convinced regarding its validity.

Note: I have NO financial or other ties with Truerife whatsoever! We sell the machines AT COST to our patients and

We have also released a NEW video / Lyme Protocols from Truerife: (if you are reading the e-book, simply click on the links. If you are reading the PRINT version of this book, go to our website to view the videos under the Lyme tab: www.upperroomwellness.com)

Click here: Lyme Protocols - YouTube for which programs to run.

Click here: Lyme Programs - YouTube NEW 2012 video from the conference!

More Video's:

Click here: Lyme Disease Experience 2011.wmv - YouTube

Click here: Rife Machines and Lyme Disease.wmv - YouTube

From time to time we get calls from individuals who have hit a plateau in their progress with Lyme disease. This can be a result of co-infections

that need to be addressed.

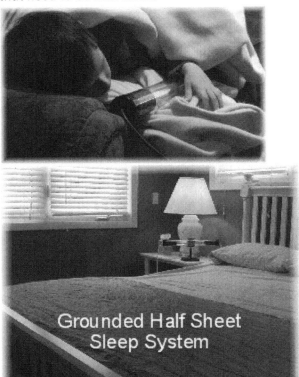

Grounded Half Sheet
Sleep System

We recommend using the Hammer Tube along with the Overnight Energy Ground Sheet to address these co-infections using the Lyme Overnight set. Our programs for patients with CLD or Cancer are created individually for them. However, those purchasing the Truerife directly from the manufacturer may utilize the Lyme sets available with great success.

A true "Rife machine", of course, is one made by Royal Rife himself. All others must be considered copycat devices, simply based on his theories but the essential understand of the Quantum Physics Rife employed is important. Rife used LIGHT frequency, so any machine NOT employing light frequency (many are electrical or sound frequency devices), though they may be beneficial, I don't consider them real Rife machines. Most of these devices are referred to as a "frequency generator" and need to legally be called experimental in nature.

One of the theories on how a Rife machine works is the principle of 'sympathetic resonance', which states that if there are two similar objects and one of them is vibrating, the other will begin to vibrate as well, even if they are not touching. Basically, if you can mimic the quantum frequency of a cell or an atom, you cause it to vibrate. This will work with sound 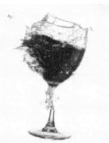 waves as well and may best be demonstrated when an opera singer hits the frequency of crystal, causing a glass to shatter. Have the atoms in the crystal changed in any way? NO, they just vibrated and were unable to remain in their current shape. The STATE of atomic structure was unaltered; the EFFECT on the atomic structure was simply mechanical. In the same way that a sound wave can induce resonance in a crystal glass and ultra-sound can be used to break up kidney stones, a Rife machine uses sympathetic resonance to physically vibrate offending cancer cells, bacteria, viruses and parasites (and YES, CLD spirochetes) resulting in their destruction and elimination from the body by causing them to virate and stimulating an immune response against them.

Another theory of illness and disease and one that may explain why Rife technology is so successful, states that since every cell of the body, from a quantum physics perspective, resonates at specific frequencies, CLD spirochetes (as well as any other pathogen) causes a dis-resonance and sets up what could be called, "low-energy" conditions in the body. Perhaps the frequency energy absorbed from a Rife machine may simply be sufficient to re-energize the body's healing capabilities, or better stated, the Rife machine, used at frequencies of specific organs or tissues, re-energizes or re-sets normal resonant frequencies and allows the body to heal itself.

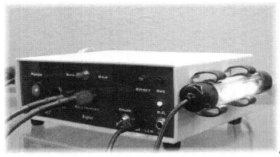
A Truerife 117 machine

Is it safe?
YES. Rife is non-invasive in the sense that the skin is not broken and there is no damage to normal, healthy tissues and cells etc. The frequencies and voltages are purposely in the range that only are harmful to cancer cells, bacteria, viruses, parasites, etc., and not healthy tissue or bacteria. Rife is non-toxic (little or no side effects other than the *standard kill-off effect*, i.e. "Herxheimer reaction", caused by any modality that destroys pathogens and necessitates the body having to clean up and detoxify the mess. This is a well-known and documented effect of any treatment that actually works. It has no ionizing radiation and so cannot cause damage to tissue, the immune system, DNA breakage, etc.)

Can I use it with other treatments?
YES. Rife can be used synergistically with most other treatment protocols (including medicine) without the danger of harmful interactions as is the case with drug therapy.

What does Rife technology work to combat?
Rife is MOST effective in dealing with microbial-based diseases (bacteria, viruses, fungi, mold, and parasites) and your own cells (cancer). It is also very beneficial to re-set normal cell frequencies. This is why patients have used the Truerife for everything from acne to hormone balance. We include over 900 pre-set programs that we and others have developed that aide patients with a wide variety of

disorders and ailments.

Is this Machine all I need?
We've seen Rife machine sessions work seemingly miraculous results –
even with cancer patients who were told (by Mayo) that they had less
than 2 weeks to live! However, we strongly believe that through diet,
supplementation, cleansing, oxygenating, and clean water, you can
dramatically improve the performance of the Rife machine and greatly
reduce your recovery time.

How long before I see results?
Everyone is different! I tell everyone that if you are looking for a "Get
Healthy Quick" scheme, look somewhere else – because with Lyme and
Cancer, there isn't one. Don't believe anyone telling you otherwise! I
believe that the MORE SPECIFIC one gets in the frequencies that will
HELP YOU, the better the results we get. This is why we SCAN all our
patients to develop their SPECIFIC PROGRAMS.

What does the equipment cost? Am I getting what I am paying for?
All of our Lyme programs and Cancer programs INCLUDE the cost of the
Rife (you will OWN it). Alone, a Rife from Truerife is $4200.

**(more detailed scientific data on Rife may be found at
http://johnbedini.net/john34/rife.html, Energy Science Forum)**

Appendix:

Helpful handouts we use in the office

The Liver Gallbladder FLUSH

The liver is an essential organ of detoxification and performs over 700 functions, far more than any other organ in the body. We cannot be healthy or recover from illness without a strong, clean well-functioning liver. If the liver is unable to carry out its full function, not only does it become congested and weak; all other organs will be more challenged as a result.

This is a liver/gallstone flush to do at home. This flush can be done in just 24 hours, so it is easy to fit into a busy schedule. It is recommended that you have done a full 7-day cleanse prior to this flush, mainly to take the toxic pressure off your organs and to be sure that your body is alkaline.

For about 5-6 days before the cleanse, it is important to **avoid fried and fatty foods** so your liver is not over-worked or stressed. **Avoid avocado, dairy, nuts and fatty meats for at least 5 to 6 days before this cleanse.** If you work a normal Monday – Friday work week, it is best to plan to do this cleanse on **Friday night (avoiding fatty foods from Sunday to that Friday),** that way you have the entire weekend to rest, relax and recover.

If you release many visible stones (yes, look in the toilet) in the first flush, it is recommended that you repeat the cleanse again in 6-8 weeks and then maybe once or twice a year.

Ingredients

- Epsom salts (Magnesium Sulfate): 4 tablespoons. *(You can usually buy this at your local pharmacy.)*

- Olive oil: 1/2 cup or 125 ml (light olive oil is easier to get down).

- Fresh pink grapefruit: 1 large or 2 small, enough to squeeze 1/2 cup (125 ml) juice. (Or use 7-8 fresh lemons/limes: squeezed into 1/2 cup juice)

- Jar or water bottle with lid – must be able to hold at least 3 cups to hold Epsom salt/water solution.

- Jar with lid (pint sized jelly jar works well) to mix olive oil/juice drink

1. **Preparation** - On Sunday through Friday, eat a diet high in alkaline-forming foods (veggies) and low in fats for at least 5 days before the cleanse. Help to gently prepare the liver by having three glasses of apple juice (preferably organic) every day for this week prior to the cleanse. Apple juice helps to dissolve the stones.

I also suggest eating beets every day during this time as well, but be warned: your BM and urine will appear red/purple.

Again, choose a day like Friday or Saturday for the cleanse, since you will be able to rest the next day. Eat a no-fat breakfast and lunch such as cooked cereal, fruit, fruit juice, bread and preserves or honey (no butter or milk). This allows the bile to build up and develop pressure in the liver. Higher pressure pushes out more stones.

2. On the morning of the cleanse, prepare the following formula below.

3. **Mix** 4 Tablespoons of Epsom Salts and 3 cups water in your water container. Mark it off to separate it into 4 equal sections

to know how much to drink each time (3/4 cup per time). Set the jar/container in the refrigerator to get cold (this is for convenience and taste only).

4. **2:00 PM.** Do not eat or drink after 2 o'clock. If you break this rule you could feel quite ill later.

5. **6:00 PM.** Drink one serving (¾ cup) of the Epsom salts/water drink. If you did not prepare this ahead of time, mix 1 tbs. in ¾ cup water now. You may add 1/8 tsp. vitamin C powder or 1/4 fresh lemon squeezed to improve the taste. You may also drink a few mouthfuls of water afterwards or rinse your mouth.

6. **8:00 PM.** Repeat by drinking another ¾ cup (185 ml) of Epsom salts and water drink. Get ready for bedtime. The timing is critical for success.

7. **9:45 PM.** Pour ½ cup (measured) olive oil into the pint jar. Squeeze the citrus fruit (fresh grapefruit, lime or lemon) by hand into the measuring cup. Remove pulp with fork. You should have at least ½ cup. Add this to the olive oil. Close the jar tightly with the lid and shake hard until watery. Do not drink it yet!

8. Now visit the bathroom one or more time, even if it makes you late for your ten o'clock drink. Don't be more than 15 minutes late. You will get fewer stones.

9. **10:00 PM.** Drink the potion you have mixed. Take it all to your bedside if you want, but drink it standing up. Get it down within 5 minutes (fifteen minutes for very elderly or weak persons).

10. **Lie down immediately**. You might fail to get stones out if you don't. The sooner you lie down the more stones you will get out. Be ready for bed ahead of time. Don't clean up the kitchen. As soon as the drink is down walk to your bed and lie down on your **right side** with your knees pulled up close to your chest.

Try to think about what is happening in the liver. Try to keep perfectly still for at least 20 minutes. You may feel a train of stones traveling along the bile ducts like marbles. There is no pain because the bile duct valves are open (thank you Epsom salts!). Go to sleep, you may fail to get stones out if you don't. Try to sleep in this position.

11. **Next morning.** Upon awakening, take your third dose of the Epsom salts and water drink. If you have indigestion or nausea wait until it is gone before drinking the Epsom salts. You may go back to bed. Don't take this potion before 6:00 am.

12. **8:00 am** (2 Hours Later) Take your fourth (the last) dose of the Epsom salts and water. You may go back to bed again.

13. After 2 More Hours you may eat. Start with fruit juice (see note below). Half an hour later eat fruit (see note below). One hour later you may eat regular food but keep it light. By supper you should feel recovered.

*NOTE – Fresh apple juice is the best juice to break the fast. At 10:00am, make fresh apple juice using 5-6 large apples in a juicer or blender and drink it. The apple juice helps dissolve gallstones and is a nice transition for the liver from the detox back to normal eating. After 30 minutes, prepare a chopped apple salad or a plain apple smoothie using 3-4 apples (with the skin is okay). If feeling unwell, stay with apples and apple juice for the entire day and only transition to light foods, salads and regular eating when you are feeling good again.

How well did you do? Expect diarrhea in the morning. Use a flashlight to look for gallstones in the toilet with the bowel movement. Look for the green kind since this is proof that they are genuine gallstones, not food residue. Only bile from the liver is pea green. The bowel movement sinks but gallstones often float because of the cholesterol inside. The first cleanse may rid you of them for a few days, but as the stones from the rear travel forward, they give you the same symptoms again. You may repeat cleanses at two week intervals. Never cleanse when you are [acutely] ill.

Sometimes the bile ducts are full of cholesterol crystals that did not form into round stones. They appear as "chaff" floating on top of the toilet bowl water. It may be tan colored, harboring millions of tiny white crystals. Cleansing this chaff is just as important as purging stones.

How safe is the liver cleanse? It is very safe. However, it can make you feel quite ill for one or two days afterwards, although in every one of these cases the maintenance parasite program had been neglected. If you have severe, acute pain, I must recommend that you check into an ER.

You may also accompany this cleanse with castor oil packs over the liver/gallbladder area.

No Gallbladder???? Here's a solution... (but make sure Dr. Conners tests you on these)

1. Your 'fattiest' meal should be between 10am and 2pm. That is when your liver produces the most bile and since you have no gallbladder to store the bile, you need to eat your fats around this time. Remember, bile is the product made by the liver to digest fats. If the bile does not have fat to bind to it when the liver secretes it, it becomes an irritant and causes a fast transit time (diarrhea).
2. GastroVen (PRL) tea helps a lot – open two capsules of GastroVen into a cup of tea (peppermint works well but use a tea flavor of choice). Sip a cup of this with each meal.
3. Digestase (PRL) – take 2 capsules per meal, with your food.
4. HCL (PRL) – take 1-2 capsules after every meal.
5. BiliVen or Gallbladder ND (PRL) - even though there is no gallbladder, the real problem was (before the gallbladder was removed) was that the bile did not flow through the bile ducts and the sluggish gallbladder and these products will help the

liver/bile from precipitating.

6. Limonene (PRL) is orange oil extract. It acts as a surfactant and breaks up oils, fats. This helps them get easily absorbed. A person without a gall bladder has a hard time absorbing fat soluble vitamins. Take 2-3 drops (in 1oz water) per meal. You can take a little more if it is a particularly fatty meal.

7. Galactan (PRL) - 1 TBL 2x per day in 8oz of water. Arabinogalactan is an immune-supporting fiber and a probiotic GI support. It will add soft bulk to the stool and stop the diarrhea.

CASTOR OIL PACKS

Following information from www.earthclinic.com:

Description:

A castor oil pack is placed on the skin to increase circulation and to promote elimination and healing of the tissues and organs underneath the skin. It is used to stimulate the liver, relieve pain, increase lymphatic circulation, reduce inflammation, and improve digestion...

Castor oil packs are made by soaking a piece of flannel in castor oil and placing it on the skin. The flannel is covered with a sheet of plastic, and then a hot water bottle is placed over the plastic to heat the pack...

Uses:

A castor oil pack can be placed on the following body regions:

The right side of the abdomen to stimulate the liver; inflamed and swollen joints, bursitis, and muscle strains; the abdomen to relieve constipation and other digestive disorders; the lower abdomen in cases of menstrual irregularities and uterine and ovarian cysts..."

Contraindications:

Do not take castor oil internally or apply to skin that is broken.

Do not use castor oil during pregnancy, breastfeeding or during menstrual flow.

Materials:

- 3 Layers of un-dyed wool or cotton flannel large enough to cover the affected area

- Castor oil

- Plastic wrap cut 1-2" larger than the flannel (can be cut from a plastic bag)

- Hot water bottle

- Container with lid

- Old clothes and sheets. Castor oil will stain clothing and bedding.

Directions:

Place the flannel in the container. Soak flannel in castor oil so that it is saturated, but not dripping. Place the pack over the affected body part. Cover with plastic. Place the hot water bottle over the pack. Leave it on for 45-60 minutes, being sure to rest while the pack is in place. After removing the pack, cleanse the area with a dilute solution of water and baking soda. Store the pack in the covered container in the refrigerator. Each pack may be reused up to 25-30 times.

Frequency:

It is generally recommended that a castor oil pack be used for 3-7 days in a week to treat a health condition or for detoxification.

Medi-Body Pack/Magma Mud Instructions

Important Note: Please read through the instructions thoroughly before using the Medi-Body/Magma Packs on any part of the body. These packs are very powerful and you may experience unnecessary detox reactions if all steps are not followed carefully.

Staining from the Medi-Body Pack™:

The Medi-Body/Magma Pack contains 100% natural ingredients and will not stain the skin or hair. However, it may stain clothing or bedding. Therefore, it's best to wear old clothes when using the Packs, and apply them outside or in the shower for easy clean-up.

Preparation:

For Medi-Body Pack: For every 2 tablespoons of **Medi-Body Pack** powder you want to add 1 capsule of HCL (open capsule and pour out contents) with approximately 2 teaspoons of the recommended liquid from your practitioner.

The **Medi-Magma** needs NO additional HCL.

Mix well in a nonmetallic container (like a glass bowl) with a nonmetallic spoon (preferably a small rubber spatula.) The consistency should be like cake batter. If you can "pour" the mixture, it's too thin. You may add more powder or liquid until the consistency is right.

The amount of mud you'll need to mix depends on the amount of sites you'll be packing. The recipe using approximately 2 tablespoons of the clay to about 2 teaspoons liquid should be enough for 3 to 4 target sites. When packing the entire hands or feet you will need to start with at least 3+ tablespoons of powder clay. It is fine to keep adding clay powder and liquid until the right amount is achieved. Just remember, for the Medi-body Pack, - for every 2 tablespoons of powder, you want to add 1capsule of HCL.

Amount of packs in one day: Remember, this is very powerful. Typically, we recommend no more than two sessions in one day. **It is NOT better to do more.** All detoxing must go slow!

Typical size of a target area: Excluding your hands and feet, the size of your target area should be no larger than the palm of your hand or the size of a tennis ball. *If a scar is longer than 6 inches, divide the scar into sections and pack 3 inches at a time. In this case, you'll need to rinse after each 3 inch section.*

Application: After selecting the target site to treat, mentally divide this area into smaller areas, each about the size of the palm of your hand. Apply only enough mud to thinly cover the first area. Rubbing the mud into the area for about 3 seconds can aid the treatment site even more. Next repeat this process on the 2nd "palm of your hand" area, etc. until you have treated all of the smaller areas of the entire target area. Then you may move on to the next target area. Once you have finished the third target area you rest with the mud in place for 15-45 minutes before you rinse.

Hands and Feet: *When packing the hands and feet the consistency of the mud should be a little more liquid.* This will allow the mud to spread evenly without drying too quickly. For the hands start at the wrists and cover the entire hand top and bottom (this includes in between the fingers) and end by rubbing into the palm vigorously. Wait 15-30 minutes before rinsing. For the feet, start at the ankles and cover the entire foot top and bottom (this includes in between the toes) to the sole. There you should rub vigorously to finish. Wait 15-30 minutes before rinsing. If you are doing both hands and feet together, pack all 4 and wait 15-30 minutes before rinsing. *Your hands and feet contain hundreds of meridian points, therefore it is very important to cover the entire area and for even better results- rub at each silver-dollar size area AND/OR set feet on an infrared-stone heating pad.*

Timing of the Packs: Generally it is best to use the Packs before 7 p.m. After this time the body begins to go into resting mode and detoxification is often more superficial. The most desirable time is in the morning or afternoon. It may make sense to do the packs before your morning shower.

Minimizing detox symptoms: Drink ½-1 tsp AloeDetox mixed with 1 cup purified water. The aloe dramatically promotes elimination of released toxins and helps prevent re-absorption.

VERY IMPORTANT NOTE: Always finish each mudpack session with a Medi Blast (foot soak). This is a crucial step that must not be skipped. The body has released toxins internally and the foot soaks will draw these toxins out.

How to do a foot soak:

Simply use a small washtub large enough for your feet. Add warm water and one of the following:

- **2 Tablespoons of Medi-Body Bath/Pack**

- **OR 1 Tablespoon Dragonite**

- **OR 1 Tablespoon 8% Food-Grade Hydrogen Peroxide**

- **OR 4 Tablespoons Epsom Salts**

**Usually Dr. Conners wants you to rotate through each of the above

***If you are using the Ion Pro Wave with your Rife, that could be done on a different day

Notes:

_____

_____

_____

_____

_____

_____

_____

_____

Where to Use Mud Packs:

1. Mudpacking Downloads – your 'downloads' are considered your hands and feet. We describe above how to do this but it is important to understand that this is how energy is taken in and released. Packing your hands/feet on a regular basis – maybe weekly while trying to get better and then monthly as a preventative measure may be helpful.

2. Trauma Points – different injuries/traumas can cause what is known as an interference field, i.e. they can block meridian energy flow in your body and prevent healing to a distant organ.

It is very common to find these interference fields and that they contribute to all sorts of diseases. Packing these help break that blockage of energy. Below is a schematic of the ones we found and homework for you:

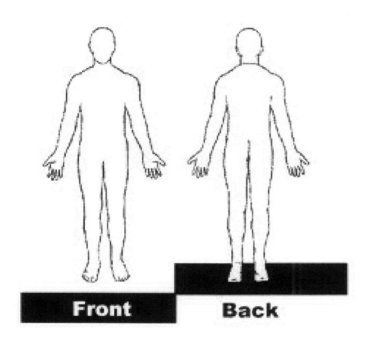

Front   **Back**

3. Organ Points – to help release toxins from an organ, help an organ/tissue heal, and/or help move block lymph, Organ Points can be packed along with the associated organ point on the feet:

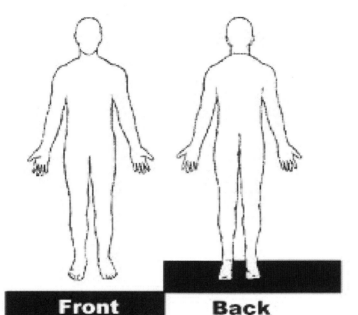

Front **Back**

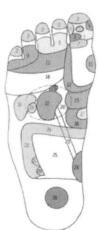

Right bottom
1. Head, left half
2. Frontal sinuses, left half
3. Brain Stem
4. Pituitary
5. Temple
6. Nose
7. Neck
8. Left Eye
9. Left Ear
11. Right Trapezoid Muscle
12. Thyroid Gland
13. Parathyroid Gland
14. Lungs, right
15. Stomach
16. Duodenum
17. Pancreas
18. Liver
19. Gall Bladder
20. Solar Plexus
21. Adrenal Gland, right
22. Kidney, right
23. Ureter, right
24. Bladder
25. Small Intestine
26. Appendix
27. Ileocecal Valve
28. Ascending colon
29. Transverse colon
36. Ovary or testicle, right

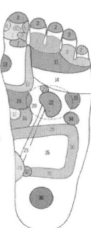

Left Bottom
1. Head, right half
2. Frontal sinuses, right half
3. Brain Stem
4. Pituitary
5. Temple
6. Nose
7. Neck
8. Right Eye
9. Right Ear
11. Left Trapezoid Muscle
12. Thyroid Gland
13. Parathyroid Gland
14. Lungs, left
15. Stomach
16. Duodenum
20. Solar Plexus
21. Adrenal Gland, left
22. Kidney, left
23. Ureter, left
24. Bladder
25. Small intestine
29. Transverse colon
30. Descending colon
31. Rectum
32. Anus
33. Heart
34. Spleen
36. Ovary or Testicle, left

4. Embedded energy blockages – these are similar to Trauma
   Points but can be worse as energy is not only blocked at the site
   but it cycles there. We still pack them but like to pack the
   special acupuncture point on the bottom of the foot to help the
   detox process. It is VERY helpful to use an Infrared heat pack
   over the points on the bottom of the feet with the mudpack:

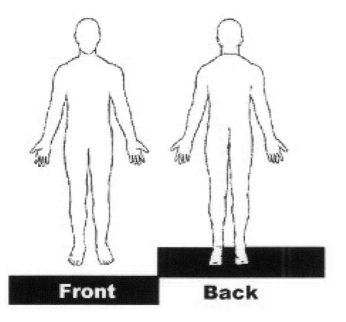

Front   **Back**

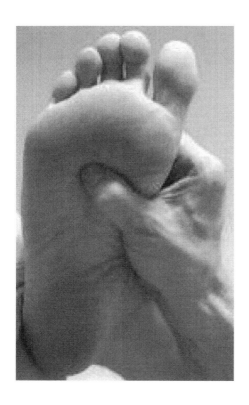

WHY ARE YOU CONSTIPATED AND WHAT CAN YOU DO ABOUT IT - Dr. Conners

The autonomic nervous system is the part of the nervous system that controls bodily functions that we do not consciously think about (think automatic functions are controlled by autonomics). For example , blood pressure, heart rate, blood flow, sweating, body temperature regulation, sleep/wake cycles, blood sugar regulation and metabolism, hormone regulation and digestion , including gut motility also known as PERISTALSIS

The autonomic nervous system is broken down into two parts: The parasympathetic and the sympathetic portions.

The parasympathetics are the part of the autonomic nervous system that keeps the bodily functions going when the body is NOT in the alarm or stressed state. The sympathetic nervous "kicks in" when we are in a stressed or alarmed state. For example, exercise or any physical endeavor, hidden FEARS, and relational stresses fire-up the sympathetic nervous system.

The parasympathetics promote peristalsis or gut motility and the sympathetics inhibit peristalsis (think about it, you don't want your bowels moving during a physical endeavor!).

When our body is not in an alarmed or stressed state our sympathetic nervous system (also known as our "fight or flight" nervous system) always needs to be inhibited or kept under control. For the most part it is our frontal lobes of the brain that do this.

Many patients with chronic illness have poor frontal lobe activation due to underlying metabolic disorders and therefore, are lacking the inhibition to the sympathetic nervous system. They live in a state of "high sympathetic tone" and suffer the symptoms of such a state. These symptoms can vary from person to person but the common ones are: migraine headaches, sensitivity to light and sound, vertigo and balance disorders, insomnia, poor blood sugar regulation and thus weight gain and fatigue, hormone imbalances, high blood pressure, anxiety, panic attacks, depression, problems breathing, frequent urination and urinary tract infections, chronic pain and CONSTIPATION .

Part of your treatment is to identify and remove the metabolic factors causing poor frontal lobe activation and to stimulate the side of the weak frontal lobe with brain based therapies (interactive metronome, eye exercises, oxygen etc...) and thus remove the state of "high sympathetic tone".

In the meantime, activation of the parasympathetics will go a long way in improving gut motility and constipation. This is done by activating cranial nerve X or the Vagus nerve which lies in your lower brain stem (the Medulla Oblongata) and controls much of gut motility. Here are a few things to do at home:

- GARGLING with warm water, HUMMING, GAGGING (with the back end of your toothbrush), SWALLOWING water .

- These activities should be done for 60-90 seconds in the morning and at night. Humming and swallowing can be done throughout the day.

- In addition, magnesium, Dr. Schulz Formula One, Dr. Christopher's Formula One, Smooth Move Tea, and others may be recommended as a short term solution.

Of course there are non-neurological reasons a person may be constipated but the results are all the same – you will re-absorb toxins! This is one reason for doing coffee enemas. Coffee enemas flush out both the intestinal tract and the liver.

One thing is certain – we do NOT want you to be constipated! Make sure you contact me if you are/become constipated.

How to Make your Own Liposomal Nutrients

Dr. Kevin Conners

www.UpperRoomWellness.com

The biggest problem with any nutrient consumption is getting the nutrient across the barriers - absorption, across the gut; across the blood-brain barrier if a needed nutrient for the brain; and across the cell membrane.

I've spoken elsewhere at length about minerals needing to be bound to an amino acid, but how about other nutrients? One way is to create nano-particles from the nutrient. Premier Research Labs does a great job of nano-izing whole-food nutrients and this is one reason that I love their products. Another way to aide barrier-crossing is to wrap it in a fat – you can even do this with the nano-ized products to improve their absorption even MORE. That is known as a liposomal particle and can be done at home with an inexpensive instrument called an ultrasonic jewelry cleaner. (Available at amazon.com for about $26.00 - http://www.amazon.com/Kendal-Digital-Ultrasonic-Cleaner-Jewelry/dp/B0001GOPZ4/ref=sr_1_10?s=jewelry&ie=UTF8&qid=1361286706&sr=1-10&keywords=ultrasonic+cleaner

Here are the steps for the Glutathione FORMULA I've developed:

1. Take 1 cups of pure water and add to a blender (I use a magic-bullet-like blender that isn't super-high speed. You do NOT want to blend it all frothy!)

2. Add 1 ½ Tablespoons of Glutathione from Designs for Health

3. Add 5 Tablespoons of Powdered Lecithin from Premier Research Labs

4. Add 4 capsules (opened and dumped in) NeuroVen from Premier Research Labs (if recommended by Dr. C)

5. Blend for 60 seconds

6. Pour mixture into Ultrasonic Cleaner and stir for 8 minutes

7. Pour into a pint-sized jar with a sealable lid

8. Store in the refrigerator

9. Shake before use and take as directed (usually 1-3 T/day)

10. You CAN throw the mixture back into the jewelry cleaner after a couple days to re-wrap it if desired

Beating Chronic LYME

Chapter Five

My Personal Philosophy

"I have told you these things, so that in me you may have peace. In this world you will have trouble. But take heart! I have overcome the world."

John 16:33

Lord, Deliver Us From EVIL

"The Spirit of the Sovereign Lord is on me, because the Lord has anointed me to proclaim good news to the poor. He has sent me to bind up the brokenhearted, to proclaim freedom for the captives and release from darkness for the prisoners" Isaiah 61:1

Freedom from demonic strongholds

I wrote this little booklet to help you gain freedom from demonic strongholds that are destroying your life. Even if you are a believer, and I might add, especially if you are a believer, the enemy will do everything possible to destroy you, your witness, your family, and your life. Quite possibly, the greatest weapon of the enemy in the believer's life is to keep him/her weak, impotent from doing anything great in the kingdom, lukewarm, selfish and carnal – all perfectly acceptable and even expected in the American Christian culture.

I wish for you to become bold, take ground back from your enemy and become strong in the Lord, filled with His Spirit to do great things. In doing so you must be ready for the battle.

If you are NOT a believer, the truth contained herein will be blinded to you. Ask God to open your eyes and give you the ability to believe. Pray a prayer similar to this, from the heart, in your own words:

"God, I don't know you. I need help. Please give me the power to believe; break the scales from my eyes; change me, mold me, shape me. I don't want religion; I want a reality with you. Make me your child; fill me with your love, your Spirit, your truth. Bind me to YOU and You alone through Your Son Jesus Christ. Give me faith. Thank you Lord."

Becoming a follower of Christ is the start. The fear of the Lord is the BEGINNING of all wisdom; it is the first step to an eternal relationship with our Creator. He desires us to commune with Him, depend on Him, and obey His voice. This requires us to KNOW His voice and we learn how to do so by learning about Him through His WORD.

Learn to LOVE the Word of God. Ask God to BIND you to His Word, bind you to a desire for His Word and a hunger for His Word. Ask him to reveal Himself to you through His Word. Discipline yourself to study, read, meditate on and memorize scripture. Be diligent to show yourself approved. This booklet is not on the spiritual disciplines but this one cannot be over-emphasized.

Walking in Obedience

As we understand Scripture, God's desire in a believer's life is to transform us into the image of His Son in a process called sanctification. This is a life-long process and different for every Christian. The Bible is also clear that we are to walk in obedience, forgiveness and love, displaying the fruits of the Spirit that can only be displayed when we are dependent on Christ and the Holy Spirit, for there is no power over our flesh or our enemy outside of the Holy Spirit as long as we are yielded to Him.

The book of Deuteronomy explains the blessings and curses assigned to God's people that promise great things to those who heed God's Word. This is **not** prosperity theology and God has never promised ease and luxury to His followers. On the contrary, Jesus warned us that, "These things I have spoken unto you, that in me ye might have peace. In the world ye shall have tribulation." We live in a fallen world system, cursed by sin and under condemnation. That is WHY we need a savior! Jesus continued completing the same verse in John, "but be of good cheer; **I** have **overcome** the **world**." (John 16:33)

It is **only** through Christ that we can overcome the world, the enemy and even ourselves. While we were yet sinners Christ died for us (Romans 5:8), taking on the punishment that we deserved, the just curse of sin. Paul stated in his letter to the Galatians, "Christ hath redeemed us from the **curse** of the law, being made a **curse** for us," dying on the cross and taking the penalty for sin.

This is the "Good News" of Scripture! We deserved death and God Himself took it upon Himself. Hallelujah! What God had done, 2000 years ago through His Son Jesus Christ, allows me to receive eternal life – forgiven and accepted as Christ. THAT is Good News!

Salvation (the above fact) and sanctification are two different things. We may be 'saved' but we still live in a fallen world, have temptations that will lead us to sin, struggle with health, finances, pain, family problems and every other issue this world, our flesh and the enemy has to throw at us – but we are not condemned. We may be beaten up and left to die physically, but spiritually we will always be bound to Christ.

However, even though we may be on our way to heaven when we die, there are things that we are called to do to protect us from this world that is always trying to attack us in various ways. Remember, God is sovereign and allows everything for our good, **but He allows some things simply because we are not being obedient to Scripture and WE are 'opening a doorway' for attack that should never have been opened.**

A simple example would be if a believer continued in a known sin while expecting God's blessings. Sanctification does NOT mean that we walk perfectly; we all sin! It DOES mean that we are to be OBEDIENT to scripture, daily confess our sin, and ask for the Holy Spirit's power over it. We are to stop doing things that lead us into sin, and get accountability from other believers so as to keep from it.

If a believer continues in a known sin regularly and unrepentively, they are really putting themselves *under a curse* and driving a wedge in their relationship with God. They are opening a doorway for Satan and his demons to enter, harass, torment, make sick, and ultimately destroy.

While the believer may still be 'saved' they will be less useful in the Kingdom, have less power to serve, become ill, aggravated, and numerous other negative manifestations bent towards the enemy's three main objectives: to steal, kill, and destroy!

For a believer to knowingly continue in sin (including a lukewarm relationship with Christ) is disobedience! Plain and simple, you were called to become an obedient child and NOT to remain foolish and ignorant regarding Spiritual things. I fully understand that though our works have *nothing* to do with salvation they have much to do with "fighting the good fight" here on earth and walking obediently with our God!

Believers may suffer things in this world for several reasons including simple effects of poor choices (overweight due to overeating, financial hardship due to slothfulness), God is allowing suffering to drive us to Him (breaking my pride, as in Paul asking three times for God to remove his problem to hear God say "My grace is sufficient for you"), God allows my suffering for His glory (as in the blind man in John 9:1-5). We can also suffer due to our **ignorance** in curses and enemy attacks.

Open Doorways

In this text, we shall refer to an "open doorway" as an entrance point for enemy attack on our life. This short treatise on the subject is in no way meant to be an exhaustive explanation of demonology and the believer's protection but rather a small introduction, a handbook to help you through recovery. In the back of this text you will find various books that we recommend; please read them and study for yourself –your life may very well depend on it!

Again, we are NOT talking about salvation! Believers, on their way to heaven when they die, can open doorways (created ignorantly by oneself, by known sin, by inherited sin, and even by others attempting to harm you) to demonic influence. Later in this booklet, I'll give you simple, child-like ways to pray against these open doorways and curses, but let's list several, simply as examples, below:

- Any past/present dealings with the occult or occult practices, no matter how lightly or briefly can become an open doorway.
- Sexual sins, including 'simple lust', pornography, dirty joke, etc.
- Idolatry, i.e. anything you spend more time thinking about than the Lord, including your position, your appearance, your success, and your ministry
- Addictions
- Involvement in Eastern Religions
- Involvement in Apostate Religions and practices
- Involvement in witchcraft, magic, voodoo, hexes, spells, psychics, mind-reading, etc.
- Involvement in Free Masonry
- Ancestral sins
- Viewing occult movies, ungodly music, TV shows, horror movies, video games displaying wrong behavior, books

that and other media that makes 'wrong' appear 'right', viewing sinful behavior of others, etc.

- Practices involving "blanking out one's mind" or "clearing one's mind" as in ungodly meditation (Godly meditation is *active* – reading the Word, studying Scripture, and memorizing verses), Yoga, TM, etc.
- Hypnosis
- Foolish talk about ourselves ("I'm so stupid, I'll never be good at that..."),
- Foolish talk about others (we can curse our loved ones, spouse or children – "my wife is a horrible cook", "my son is lazy"...),
- Other, well-meaning relations cursing us (parent, teacher, pastor saying untrue statements),
- Evil prayers (curses) of unsaved people attempting to hurt us (any nasty comment maligning your character that isn't edifying for correction), and even ancestral curses (a father involved in occult practices).

In our office, we deal with many very sick patients and though I know that ALL of us are going to die, sometimes we suffer needlessly from chronic illness linked to curses and open doorways allowing demonic activity such as those listed above. Of course it isn't all the time, but praying correctly as I list below is simply the right thing to do.

"If we confess our sins, He is faithful and just to forgive us our sins, and to cleanse us from all unrighteousness." 1 John 1:9

Example Prayer to Close Doorways:

"Father, I confess to you my involvement in _____. I now recognize that such a thing is an abomination to you and detestable in your sight. I humbly ask your forgiveness and ask that you lift out any demonic entrance as a result of my actions and that you cleanse me and close any and all doorways I have opened. Please close these open

doorways and cleanse me in the precious blood of Jesus, in Jesus name I ask, Amen."

Then take authority over your life:

"Satan and you demons, I have asked my heavenly Father for forgiveness for participating in _____ and have received His mercy! I now, by faith in what God has already done through Jesus Christ, close that doorway to you, now and forever, through the blood of Jesus. Now, in Jesus name, get away from me!

We are called to 'fight the good fight' and 'finish the race' and should desire, more than anything else, to hear our Savior say, "Well done good and faithful servant... come and enter into rest and joy of the Lord." (Matthew 25:21)

It might be a good idea to do a word study on Blessings and Curses. Below are some passages that may be helpful to recite regularly if you struggle with health issues:

Psalm 118:17-29: "[17]I shall not die, but live, and declare the works of the LORD.

[18]The LORD hath chastened me sore: but he hath not given me over unto death.

[19]Open to me the gates of righteousness: I will go into them, and I will praise the LORD:

[20]This gate of the LORD, into which the righteous shall enter.

[21]I will praise thee: for thou hast heard me, and art become my salvation.

[22]The stone which the builders refused is become the head stone of the corner.

²³This is the LORD's doing; it is marvelous in our eyes.

²⁴This is the day which the LORD hath made; we will rejoice and be glad in it.

²⁵Save now, I beseech thee, O LORD: O LORD, I beseech thee, send now prosperity.

²⁶Blessed be he that cometh in the name of the LORD: we have blessed you out of the house of the LORD.

²⁷God is the LORD, which hath shewed us light: bind the sacrifice with cords, even unto the horns of the altar.

²⁸Thou art my God, and I will praise thee: thou art my God, I will exalt thee.

²⁹O give thanks unto the LORD; for he is good: for his mercy endureth forever."

James 4:7 – " ⁷Submit yourselves therefore to God. Resist the devil, and he will flee from you."

Ephesians 1:3-9 – "³Blessed be the God and Father of our Lord Jesus Christ, who hath blessed us with all spiritual blessings in heavenly places in Christ:

⁴According as he hath chosen us in him before the foundation of the world, that we should be holy and without blame before him in love:

⁵Having predestinated us unto the adoption of children by Jesus Christ to himself, according to the good pleasure of his will,

⁶To the praise of the glory of his grace, wherein he hath made us accepted in the beloved.

⁷In whom we have redemption through his blood, the forgiveness of sins, according to the riches of his grace;

⁸Wherein he hath abounded toward us in all wisdom and prudence;

⁹Having made known unto us the mystery of his will, according to his good pleasure which he hath purposed in himself."

Colossians 1:10-18 – "¹⁰That ye might walk worthy of the Lord unto all pleasing, being fruitful in every good work, and increasing in the knowledge of God;

¹¹Strengthened with all might, according to his glorious power, unto all patience and longsuffering with joyfulness;

¹²Giving thanks unto the Father, which hath made us meet to be partakers of the inheritance of the saints in light:

¹³Who hath delivered us from the power of darkness, and hath translated us into the kingdom of his dear Son:

¹⁴In whom we have redemption through his blood, even the forgiveness of sins:

¹⁵Who is the image of the invisible God, the firstborn of every creature:

¹⁶For by him were all things created, that are in heaven, and that are in earth, visible and invisible, whether they be thrones, or dominions, or principalities, or powers: all things were created by him, and for him:

¹⁷And he is before all things, and by him all things consist.

¹⁸And he is the head of the body, the church: who is the beginning, the firstborn from the dead; that in all things he might have the preeminence."

Luke 10:17-20 - "¹⁷And the seventy returned again with joy, saying, Lord, even the devils are subject unto us through thy name.

¹⁸And he said unto them, I beheld Satan as lightning fall from heaven.

¹⁹Behold, I give unto you power to tread on serpents and scorpions, and over all the power of the enemy: and nothing shall by any means hurt you.

²⁰Notwithstanding in this rejoice not, that the spirits are subject unto you; but rather rejoice, because your names are written in heaven.

Some simple steps to Walking in the Blessing regardless of your situation:

1. Recognize – the truth of fleshly, worldly, and demonic desires in your life. The devil is like a roaring lion. He and his minions desire to steal, kill and destroy all that is good - including you. Failure to recognize that you have an enemy is grounds for immediate loss. Understand that Jesus Christ has already won your 'battle' against your flesh, the world and the forces of evil. Your moment-by-moment job is to hang on tight to Him who drags us through the mess. Sin (wrong thoughts and deeds), selfishness (which is idolatry), and self-righteousness (Jesus only yelled at the religious pretenders!) MUST be confessed and repented of or you are just pretentious. There is NO room for "lukewarm" people and God will vomit them out of His mouth (see Revelation 3:14-22).

2. Repent of anything you opened to evil, past and present sin. Repentance is not an act that solely happened at a moment in the past it is a verb of the present tense where we are COMMANDED to turn from sin daily. Matthew 3; James 4:7

3. Renounce – declare that you are no longer going to be subject to these things. "I refuse it; I renounce it; it no longer has a place in my life, Lord bind me to YOU. I'm not submitting to evil any longer…" Eph 1:7, Col 1:12-14. You are going to fall – expect it. Listen, being a Christian does NOT mean that you

are not going to sin! My definition of maturity is that WHEN you Do sin, you will more quickly hear the conviction of the Holy Spirit and repent of it!

4. Resist – keep up the good fight – bind yourself to Christ, this is our 'work'. Gal 3:13-14, 1 John 3:8, Luke 10:19. Goodness sakes, it is difficult for most men to not look at a beautiful woman with a bit of lust – but it is SIN. It is difficult for most Americans to not lust for new houses, cars, or big-screen TVs. Just STOP, Apologize to God and know that you're forgiven. Not that it's wrong to want a new TV but if you are lusting after something it is an idol!

5. Confess your Faith in Christ DAILY – read Scripture aloud to yourself. Develop some system of affirmative verses that motivate you to keep on course; find others to hold you accountable who won't let you whine, wallow in self-pity, and will pick you up when you stumble.

6. Commit to obedience – hear God's voice (through His Word) and do what He says. Goodness sakes, Americans think that they're 'saved' because they prayed a prayer X amount of years ago, go to church, got baptized, were confirmed... (and maybe they are, I'm not the judge of that), BUT failure to attempt to walk in obedience to His word should be a SIGN that all things aren't well at the home front!

7. Confess any known sins daily (remember my definition of maturity). Confess known/unknown sins of ancestors. Get rid of all 'contact objects'

8. Forgive anything and everything against anyone and everyone – a HUGE stumbling block.

9. Release yourself to Jesus verbally – "Lord bind me to You".

10. Confess and expect the blessing of Abraham – the Holy Spirit gives the blessing, ask for it!

Example prayers: (it's not the words that matter most, it is your heart)

"Lord Jesus Christ, I believe that you are the Son of God and the ONLY way to God. I believe that You chose to become a curse on the cross so that I might be released from the curse and all curses against me. Lord I commit myself to your truth; please bind me to your truth and your blessing. Please reveal any and all sins I've committed and all disobedience against you in thoughts or actions, past or present, from me or placed on me; forgive me Lord, wash me clean by your blood; seal me with your Holy Spirit. Give me the power to forgive everyone that has ever wronged me, including forgiving myself, that I may fully receive your forgiveness. I renounce all contact with the occult – please reveal any connection that my attempt to bind me to anything but you. And know, having received my forgiveness by faith and with the authority of a child of the most high, I release myself and all those under my authority from any curse over our lives, asking you to bind us to your heart, to obedience to you alone, and to the receive the blessings you have promised, in the name and power of Jesus Christ. Thank you Jesus!"

Walk in this DAILY.

Acknowledgements/affirmations:

1. I acknowledge that there is an enemy, Satan and his demons, that desire that I remain sick, poor, self-focused, immature and everything bad. But I also understand that my fleshly, selfish thoughts and wrong, distorted beliefs may be even more responsible for where I am. In all things God desires to

work towards good towards those who love Him, so I know my fight is against this world, my flesh, and the enemy.

2. I acknowledge that though I have surrendered my spirit to Christ, my flesh wars against the things of God's Spirit and my daily walk of sanctification involves repentance of thoughts and deeds contrary to God's will for me. I fully understand that I can do NONE of this (victoriously) myself and that God desires to do all of it for me. My work is to completely depend on Him and walk daily in obedience.

3. I acknowledge that God has sent His Son to pay the price of my sin and has eternally conquered sin, death, and all evil and that when I am 'in Him' and His will, my spirit is protected and safe. Greater is HE that is in me than he that is in the world.

More Example Prayers:

1. "Lord, please BIND me to Your will, not mine, Your Spirit, Your Truth which is beyond my comprehension. I pray that You loose, break, destroy, crush all thoughts, beliefs and dogmas that are contrary to You and Your truth."

2. "Lord, BIND me to Your will in my life, reveal today that which You desire for me. Help me surrender and lay down my will, desires, plans and dreams. Give me new desires in my heart; bind me to them, bound to Your will, yoked to Christ, trusting wholly in You, what You have already done and what You will do in my life."

3. "Lord, open my eyes to my flesh and let me discern Your will from mine. Loose my fleshly connections with the world, give me Your heart, moment by moment."

4. "Lord, let me see others as You see them. Fill me with Your Spirit that You may pour out to them all that You desire. Bind me, swaddled like a babe is to her mother, to Your

heart, Your mind, Your love, Your mercy, Your forgiveness, Your goodness, Your patience, and Your truth."

5. "Lord, I beg that YOU be glorified in my life. Loose my fleshly ties to my 'rights' and my self-centered desires to be exalted. Loose the many idols in my heart and BIND me to You alone. Let You and Your name be glorified. Let this be my prayer for others as well, friends and enemies."

6. "Thank you Lord for EVERYTHING, even that which, in my flesh, I deemed 'bad'. Let ALL things drive me to You. Thank You that I may fully and completely depend and trust in YOU."

7. "Lord comfort me with the full knowledge of Your unbelievable love for me. Woo me in the awe of the depth, the height, and the width of Your mercy, your care, your everlasting peace for me. Loose all doubt and fear, guilt and shame, indecision, confusion, sadness and anxiety. Bind me to YOU. Thank you!"

Blessings and Curses on Our Lives

As we understand Scripture, God's desire in a believer's life is to transform us into the image of His Son in a process called sanctification. This is a life-long process and different for every Christian. The Bible is also clear that we are to walk in obedience, forgiveness and love, displaying the fruits of the Spirit that can only be displayed when we are dependent on Christ and the Holy Spirit, for there is no power over our flesh or our enemy outside of the Holy Spirit as long as we are yielded to Him.

The book of Deuteronomy explains the blessings and curses assigned to God's people that promise great things to those who heed God's Word. This is not prosperity theology and God has never promised ease and luxury to His followers. On the contrary, Jesus warned us that, "These things I have spoken unto you, that in me ye might have peace. In the world ye shall have tribulation." We live in a fallen world system, cursed by sin and under condemnation. That is WHY we need a savior! Jesus continued completing the same verse in John, "but be of good cheer; I have overcome the world." (John 16:33)

It is only through Christ that we can overcome the world, the enemy and even ourselves. While we were yet sinners Christ died for us (Romans 5:8), taking on the punishment that we deserved, the just curse of sin. Paul stated in his letter to the Galatians, "Christ hath redeemed us from the curse of the law, being made a curse for us," dying on the cross and taking the penalty for sin. This is the "Good News" of Scripture! We deserved death and God Himself took it upon Himself. Hallelujah! What God had done, 2000 years ago through His Son Jesus Christ, allows me to receive eternal life – forgiven and accepted as Christ. THAT is Good News!

Salvation (the above fact) and sanctification are two different things. We may be 'saved' but we still live in a fallen world, have temptations that will lead us to sin, struggle with health, finances, pain, family problems and every other issue this world, our flesh and the enemy has to throw at us – but we are not condemned. We may be beaten up and left to die physically, but spiritually we will always be bound to Christ.

However, even though we may be on our way to heaven when we die, there are things that we are called to do to protect us from this world that is always trying to attack us in various ways. Remember, God is sovereign and allows everything for our good, but He allows some things simply because we are not being obedient to Scripture and WE are 'opening a doorway' for attack that should never have been opened. A simple example would be if a believer continued in a known sin while expecting God's blessings. Sanctification does NOT mean that we walk perfectly; we all sin. It DOES mean that we confess our sin and ask for the Holy Spirit's power over it, stop doing things that lead us into it, and get accountability from other believers so as to keep from it. If a believer continues in a known sin daily and unrepentive they are really putting themselves under a curse and driving a wedge in their relationship with God. They still may be 'saved' but they will be less useful in the Kingdom and have less power to serve. This is disobedient and though our works have nothing to do with salvation they have much to do with "fighting the good fight" here on earth.

Believers may suffer things in this world for several reasons including simple effects of poor choices (overweight due to overeating, financial hardship due to slothfulness), God is allowing suffering to drive us to Him (breaking my pride as in Paul asking three times for God to remove his problem to hear God say "My grace is sufficient for you"), God allows my suffering for His glory (as in the blind man in John 9:1-5). We can also suffer due to our ignorance in curses. Foolish talk about ourselves ("I'm so stupid, I'll never be good at that..."), foolish talk about others (we can curse our loved ones, spouse or children – "my wife is a horrible cook", "my son is lazy"...), other, well-meaning relations cursing us (parent, teacher, pastor saying untrue statements), evil prayers (curses) of unsaved people attempting to hurt us (any nasty comment maligning your character that isn't edifying for correction), and even ancestral curses (a father involved in occult practices). Understand, these things have NO POWER over a believer unless we have given it power – which often, we unknowingly have.

We deal with many very sick patients and though I know that ALL of us are going to die, sometimes we suffer needlessly from chronic illness linked to curses such as the above. Of course it isn't all the time, but praying correctly as I list below is simply the right thing to do. We are called to 'fight the good fight' and 'finish the race' and should all desire, more than anything else to hear our Savior say, "Well done good and faithful servant... come and enter into rest and joy of the Lord." (Matthew 25:21)

It might be a good idea to do a word study on Blessings and Curses. Below are some passages that may be helpful to recite regularly if you struggle with health issues:

Psalm 118:17-29: "I shall not die, but live, and declare the works of the LORD. The LORD hath chastened me sore: but he hath not given me over unto death. Open to me the gates of righteousness: I will go into them, and I will praise the LORD: This gate of the LORD, into which the righteous shall enter. I will praise thee: for thou hast heard me, and art become my salvation. The stone which the builders refused is become the head stone of the corner. This is the LORD's doing; it is marvelous in our eyes. This is the day which the LORD hath made; we will rejoice and be glad in it. Save now, I beseech thee, O LORD: O LORD, I beseech thee, send now prosperity. Blessed be he that cometh in the name of the LORD: we have blessed you out of the house of the LORD. God is the LORD, which hath shewed us light: bind the sacrifice with cords, even unto the horns of the altar. Thou art my God, and I will praise thee: thou art my God, I will exalt thee. O give thanks unto the LORD; for he is good: for his mercy endureth forever."

James 4:7 – "Submit yourselves therefore to God. Resist the devil, and he will flee from you."

Ephesians 1:3-9 – "Blessed be the God and Father of our Lord Jesus Christ, who hath blessed us with all spiritual blessings in heavenly places in Christ. According as he hath chosen us in him before the foundation of the world, that we should be holy and without blame before him in love. Having predestinated us unto the adoption of children by Jesus Christ to himself, according to the good pleasure of his will, to the praise of the glory of his grace, wherein he hath made us accepted in the beloved. In whom we have redemption through his blood, the forgiveness of sins, according to the riches of his grace; Wherein he hath abounded toward us in all wisdom and prudence; Having made known unto us the mystery of his will, according to his good pleasure which he hath purposed in himself."

Colossians 1:10-18 – "10That ye might walk worthy of the Lord unto all pleasing, being fruitful in every good work, and increasing in the knowledge of God; Strengthened with all might, according to his glorious power, unto all patience and longsuffering with joyfulness;

Giving thanks unto the Father, which hath made us meet to be partakers of the inheritance of the saints in light, Who hath delivered us from the power of darkness, and hath translated us into the kingdom of his dear Son, In whom we have redemption through his blood, even the forgiveness of sins, Who is the image of the invisible God, the firstborn of every creature. For by him were all things created, that are in heaven, and that are in earth, visible and invisible, whether they be thrones, or dominions, or principalities, or powers: all things were created by him, and for him. And he is before all things, and by him all things consist. And he is the head of the body, the church, who is the beginning, the firstborn from the dead; that in all things he might have the preeminence."

Luke 10:17-20 - "And the seventy returned again with joy, saying, Lord, even the devils are subject unto us through thy name. And he said unto them, I beheld Satan as lightning fall from heaven. Behold, I give unto you power to tread on serpents and scorpions, and over all the power of the enemy: and nothing shall by any means hurt you. Notwithstanding in this rejoice not, that the spirits are subject unto you; but rather rejoice, because your names are written in heaven.

Final acknowledgements and nutritional supplementation/supply companies I use:

Premier Research Labs
3500 Wadley Place, Bldg. B
Austin, TX 78728 USA
http://www.prlabs.com

Designs For Health
http://www.designsforhealth.com

Apex Energetics
16592 Hale Ave.
Irvine, CA 92606
Toll Free Order: 800-736-4381
http://www.orderapex.com

Truerife
564 Fineview
Kalamazoo, MI 49004 USA
www.truerife.com

Klaire Labs
ProThera®, Inc.
10439 Double R Blvd, Reno, NV 89521
www.klaire.com

Hope Science
P.O. Box 181825
Coronado, CA 92178
www.hopescience.com

Again, NO part of this book should be used or protocols followed without the advice of your personal physician!

Contact information:

You may contact Dr. Conners at the below address. He currently accepts new patients from around the world that suffer with cancer, chronic Lyme, and chronic autoimmune disorders.

Dr. Kevin Conners
Upper Room Wellness, Inc.
1654 County Road E E
Vadnais Heights, MN 55110
www.UpperRoomWellness.com

651.739.1248

Made in the USA
Charleston, SC
23 October 2013